Her
Beautiful
Brain

Her
Beautiful
Brain

Ann Hedreen

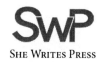

SHE WRITES PRESS

Published 2014
Printed in the United States of America
ISBN: 978-1-938314-92-6
Library of Congress Control Number: 2014934292

For information, address:
She Writes Press
1563 Solano Ave #546
Berkeley, CA 94707

There are as many versions of every family's history as there are family members. This is
mine. Some names of people and places have been changed.

To my husband, Rustin
And my mother, Arlene

CONTENTS

Prologue: Typing Class

I had a new nightmare: I was suffocating in the giant breasts of Miss Weis, as she surrounded me and contorted my fingers into unnatural positions and—from just next to my ear—yelled her commands to the class. "Ready, go! The quick brown fox jumps over the lazy dog. Faster! The quick brown fox jumps over the lazy dog. Faster! The quick brown fox . . ."

Louder and louder she shouted, as I struggled for breath, trapped inside her titanic bosom. Gone were the old dreams of giant spiders under my bed or my braces being tightened by a plumber's wrench. Miss Weis now reigned supreme over my nights, screaming about the quick brown fox and the lazy dog, predicting my doomed future: unable to get a good secretarial job, I would wander the earth in search of work as a waitress, a maid, a janitor.

It was 1969. I was twelve years old. Fall semester, eighth grade, Nathan Eckstein Junior High School, Seattle, Washington. I had no future because I could not type.

Ah, Miss Weis! You saw my clumsy fingers and you feared for me. You sized up my pointy tortoise-shell glasses and my mouth full of braces and yes, you feared for me. You knew that girls like me *had* to learn to type. You knew that all that noise about times allegedly a-changin' was just that, noise, and that your mission was to form the fingers of vulnerable girls, to train their hands, before their heads got all filled up with all this new noise about college and careers and, God forbid, Women's Lib.

Ah, Miss Weis. You gave me my first C. Maybe you grieved for me a little as you noted it in your ledger. But then you moved on to the next

1

semester: six more class periods, thirty students per period. A few boys, but you ignored them, those lazy dogs, because you knew they didn't need you. The girls needed you.

And I moved on too, like a quick brown fox, running as fast as I could from the future as envisioned by Miss Weis.

And the times, they did change. Fancy east coast colleges decided they wanted geographic diversity and public school kids, and Wellesley College gave me a scholarship.

And typewriters changed too. Correct-tape was invented, thank the Lord. Electric typewriters were now affordable, and Mom gave me a little blue Royal as a high school graduation present. And, just as Miss Weis had predicted, typing kept my body and soul together. I typed all of one summer at my grandfather's insurance company, convinced I was going crazy. But by the end of that summer I was able to type faster than I could think. At college, I typed other girls' papers for cash. After college, my first job title was "secretary" at a Boston publishing company, where I was given charge of my very own Queen of All Typewriters, the IBM Selectric. Miss Weis would have been astounded by the speeds I reached: sixty, seventy, 100 words per minute. Fingers flying, hands properly arched, off I went, typing my way into adulthood.

Just as my mom had, a quarter century earlier. Divorced, with two small children and one year at the University of Montana, it was her typing and her math skills that got her in the door at a life insurance company.

When I was twenty-one and in that first job, smarting a little every time I saw the word "secretary" next to my freshly graduated name, there was a part of me that felt defeated by the world, by the fact that I was doing exactly what my mother had done to stay alive, back in the dark ages of the early fifties. There was a part of me that felt ashamed for having taken the Little, Brown personnel director at her word when she explained that "all of our young women start as secretaries, while our young men start as sales reps." It was 1978. I should have stormed out of the office. Many of my Wellesley classmates would have. But I was paying my own rent, and I was being offered a job in publishing, and

I took it. And though it wasn't right or fair that it was the ONLY start offered me by personnel director Cindy Cool, it was a start.

A start I never would have gotten without Miss Weis and her metronome and her quick brown fox.

Fast-forward thirty-plus years, and my husband and I are walking around a little building in south Seattle called the Telephone Museum. We are there because we're making a documentary film about Alzheimer's disease, which has been hard at work destroying my mom's brain for at least a decade. We're looking for visual metaphors and they are everywhere: colorful tangles of cables, rows of big black switches with labels like Data and Memory. Then we see an old Teletype machine. We both spent most of the 1980s in newsrooms, so a Teletype evokes a visceral reaction for us, a cascade of all the events we first saw in staccato type beating down on rolls of newsprint: John Lennon murdered. Challenger exploded. Grenada invaded.

"Could you turn it on?" we ask.

"Sure," our guide, a retired phone company lifer, responds. The machine, which is the size of a snowmobile, hums to life. Then he presses the red Test button and the beautiful clacking begins, and we see the test sentence: "The quick brown fox jumps over the lazy dog." Carriage return, repeat. "The quick brown fox jumps over the lazy dog." Return, repeat. Over and over again, in twelve-point Courier type. We are hypnotized.

"Could you make it screw up?" my husband asks.

We watch as our guide hits "repeat" before the full test line is typed. The keys falter and jam. He does it again and then again. Soon, there's a pileup of a dozen keys and a black blot of text on newsprint.

Quick Brown Fox becomes the title of our film.

It wasn't obvious enough, we were told. It will hurt sales. And maybe it did. But we stuck by it. The sight of the keys jamming on an old Teletype said everything we needed to say in one image about Alzheimer's disease.

And it said more. For all the generations of women who typed to feed their children, to get through college, to survive, the words *Quick*

Brown Fox said struggle and survival. They said that this life does not deserve to end in the jammed keys and black ink of Alzheimer's disease.

Computers have put the secretaries and the Miss Weises of the world out of a job. Now, executives bend their groomed fingers around smart phones and our children type faster than we do.

But these are boom times for Alzheimer's disease.

My mother was seventy-four when she died after nearly two decades of first knowing that "something was going wrong" and then knowing that she had Alzheimer's disease. She had always planned to write her own story. Instead, her life ended wordlessly, all connections between brain and speech finally severed. Not for lack of trying: she had labored mightily to keep communicating, in English, then gibberish, then smiles and hums, just as she had tried to keep walking, feeding herself, focusing on a photo or a face, until it was as utterly impossible for her as turning on the TV when the power's out. No current means no current: you can't blow on it like a little bit of kindling and paper and make it spark.

Mom's last years were her own version of the Miss Weis nightmare, though she was suffocated not by giant breasts but by plaques and tangles that made her efforts to write or speak as useless as typing and typing while the keys tripped and jammed, the letters melting into a black puddle, the paper itself tearing from the weight of the pooling ink, nothing she wanted to say ever getting said. Her Alzheimer's disease was not a blank page; it was a sticky swamp.

I want to tell the story that I think she wanted to tell. It's her story, but it's mine too. The film we made was the first step. Now, I am sitting down at the keyboard to type. To write all that we couldn't say in the film. At least, thanks to Miss Weis, I know my fingers can keep up.

In Haiti

Twenty-three years have passed, but I can still picture my mother stepping off the plane in Port-au-Prince, her silver hair blasted by the hot Haitian wind, her nose taking in for the first time the tangled smells of overripe mangoes, a million cooking fires, rivers of sewage; the humidity triggering a tidal surge of her own sweat the likes of which she's never experienced in her temperate life. I can see her walking with the crowd from the plane, everyone around her yelling, frantically trying to find each other, find their luggage, get going, in a language she had thought would sound more like French.

She's traveling alone. She hasn't told me, or anyone, that she thinks something might be wrong with her brain.

This was my mom, Arlene Marie Grundstrom Lind Hedreen Tocantins, on the afternoon of March 31, 1987. She was fifty-six years old. Two decades later, she's gone, fully erased at last by the plaques and tangles that were already, on that spring afternoon in Haiti, wrapping tendrils around her neurons, like morning glory vines quietly going to work on a garden.

The passport in her hand that day was still shiny blue because she had only used it a few times in her life. But her youngest child of six, my baby sister Caroline, was in the Peace Corps, and Mom had promised she'd visit.

I had been in Port-au-Prince for two days when she arrived. I was a TV news producer for the CBS station in Seattle and I was producing a series of stories on Peace Corps volunteers in Haiti and the Dominican Republic. Caroline had given me the idea when she mentioned in a letter written during her fall training in Washington, D.C. that a surprising number of volunteers from Washington State had been assigned to Caribbean countries.

I knew that Haiti was the poorest country in the Western Hemisphere because I'd been doing my homework. But I thought I was pretty worldly because I had lived in England for two years, one as a student and one as a waitress, and traveled Europe on the cheap. I was looking forward to finding real croissants and café au lait in Port-au-Prince, maybe flexing a little French. I was beside myself with excitement at being out of the newsroom for two whole weeks.

I had just turned thirty and I had been officially divorced for less than a month. Traveling with me was my new boyfriend, Rus (short for Rustin), who, to the annoyance of some of the older guys, was getting a reputation as one of the best cameramen at our Seattle station. He was good-looking, too, in a young Tom Selleck way. Some people thought he was arrogant but that's because they didn't know him like I did; they didn't know that deep down, he was a class-clown movie geek who had escaped a blue-collar high school for the University of Washington. I had just spent the most romantic working week ever with Rus in the Dominican Republic and I couldn't wait to introduce him to my sister.

That was me in the spring of 1987: in the full, selfish, glorious bloom of new love, topped off by the thrill of the biggest break yet in my working life. Looking forward to dipping croissants and interviewing Peace Corps workers and hanging out with my sister, barely thinking about the fact that my mom would be there, too. Still kicking myself for not checking her schedule, for not realizing that the only week that Mom, a high school teacher, could make *her* big trip to Haiti happened to be the very same week that Rus and I would be there.

Haiti, in the spring of 1987, was also in the bloom of love: a torrid and turbulent infatuation with democracy. On the very day Rus and I arrived, March 29, 1987, Haitians had lined up at dawn to ratify their new constitution in the first free and fair election in the republic's history. Their hated dictator, "Baby Doc" Duvalier, had been banished for more than a year. People wore T-shirts proclaiming "Haiti Libérée 3 Février 1986," which was the day Duvalier was put on a plane to France. The flights coming in from Miami to Port-au-Prince were packed with well-to-do Haitians returning home with TVs and coffeemakers, their little girls in dresses that looked like wedding cakes and their little boys in tiny suits.

A white couple who resembled my southern, golf-loving former in-laws stood behind us in the passport line. They heard us talking about where to stay: the Peace Corps had not reserved anything for us, as they had in the D.R., so we were winging it. The only hotel we had heard of was the Hotel Oloffson, the setting for Graham Greene's novel, *The Comedians*.

"Excuse me," said the golf-skirted woman, in a sweet Dixie voice. "I can't help but overhear you. I believe the Oloffson is closed for repairs." She spoke calmly, as if she often had to guide people like us through their first hours in Haiti. "It's going to be hard for you to find a place, what with the election and all. Why don't you stay in our company's apartment at the Hotel Montana? We're with Stride Rite Shoes and we keep a guest apartment at the Montana. It's really the best place to stay. The safest, on a day like this."

She insisted. We looked at our cases of TV gear and agreed. Soon, we were following her swaying skirt to her four-wheel-drive Montero and then listening from the back seat as she narrated while her husband drove the car a few feet at a time through the post-election throngs of Port-au-Prince.

Stride Rite had a shoe factory in Haiti and her husband had run it for ten years. They lived in Pétionville, a suburb of Port-au-Prince, which she said was the nicest place to live because it was up in the hills and not so hot.

Outside our windows, the streets were becoming more and more jammed, the few cars and trucks swimming upstream in a river of people, wave upon wave of brown and black faces, their heads piled high with bobbing stacks of clothing and bags of rice and beans and baskets full of fruit or peanuts or live chickens; all the women wearing head scarves, some bright or white but most old and faded. The smells were of smoke and sewage and dozens of less identifiable aromas: Spoiling meat? Exotic flowers? The sounds were of vendors calling urgently, as if to make up for the time they'd lost that morning casting their votes, and the unmuffled motors and bleating horns of the tap-taps, trucks jammed with people and brightly painted with curlicues and flowers and saints and slogan-like names in Kreyol or French or English: "Baby Jesus Deliver Us," "Merci Bon Dieu."

I sat in the back seat, feeling awed and amazed and profoundly embarrassed: for not having understood the importance of the election, for having thought there would be cafés with croissants, for having craved any such thing. For having been lulled by the relative luxuries of the D.R.—where the Peace Corps had been operating for twenty-five years and could afford to assign someone to take care of our needs full-time for a week—into thinking Haiti would be more of the same.

Embarrassed, yes, but humbly on fire, too—with the fervent thrill of being in a place that I could see was unlike anywhere I'd ever been. And I was there with Rus. Whatever Haiti had in store for us, we would stumble through it together. Look at what had just happened: we'd been offered a ride and a place to stay!

It was hard to imagine Mom arriving in just a few days and having to jump into the bedlam of post-election Port-au-Prince: Mom, who had lately been oddly distracted, self-absorbed, even, as if the minutiae of her life—papers to grade, tennis to schedule, bills to pay—was so preoccupying that she couldn't retain any details about the lives of her six grownup children, let alone their spouses or new boyfriends.

The crowds thinned as we climbed up and up, out of the city and into Pétionville, where the streets were paved with river rocks in hand-laid patterns and shaded with unfamiliar trees. At the end of a lane on the highest hill stood the Hotel Montana, a white stucco palace with an electronic gate that swung open as we approached. When we pulled in, the sunset was streaking the sky like a smashed papaya mixed with soot. Far below, cooking fires and a few weak streetlights dotted the city, tiny fireflies of light compared to what you'd see from a hillside above any

North American or European city. An encouraging smell of grilled meat drifted from the hotel restaurant.

The Stride Rites handed over the key and refused any payment. "We're so happy to help," Mrs. Stride Rite said, as if it were the simplest thing in the world to open up the company apartment to two total strangers. "Haiti needs all the good publicity she can get. We're thrilled that the Peace Corps is here now and that you're doing your story."

We were tired and grateful. We had one long day of shooting ahead, before the day when Mom would arrive and Caroline would come into the city to meet us. And the apartment, which faced away from the city and toward the faded, square-cut hills of central Haiti, had two bedrooms, which would be a nice surprise for Mom and Caroline. I knew Mom had spent more than she should have on her plane ticket, and Caroline was living on practically nothing.

The next morning, as Rus and I drove away from the Hotel Montana, I began to understand why Haiti looked the way it did from the air. When you fly into Haiti from the Dominican Republic, you fly from green to brown: from the green half of the island of Hispaniola—where Columbus first set foot, planted the flag for his patrons, the King and Queen of Spain, and got to work slaughtering Taínos and Caribs—to the brown half. This was true two decades ago and—as the whole world could see in the aerial footage shot after the cataclysmic January 2010 earthquake—it is even more starkly true today. Haiti's trees are disappearing because they are the only source of cooking fuel that most Haitians can afford. The resulting erosion has turned most roads into successions of potholes that are full of dust in the dry season and mud in the rainy season. That dry-season day, we were driving deep into the dusty middle of the island to profile a veteran Peace Corps volunteer who was working in one of the poorest, barest areas.

Our driver was not much of a talker and he had to stay focused on the constant, crazy dips in the road. Our only common language was French, which neither he nor I spoke very well and Rus spoke not at all.

As we bumped silently along, my mind wandered to Mom and all the many reasons why I was not looking forward to seeing her in Haiti.

All my life, I had idolized my mother as the strong, smart survivor, the Woman of Steel. But in 1987, I was in love and she was a walking reminder of where love can leave you: in her case, divorced twice and widowed once. She was also a walking reminder that, like her first two husbands, I had behaved badly and hurt someone. *Behaved badly:* I couldn't even say that big bad word—*adultery*—the word I had hated since I was twelve, when my parents split up and I started going to a church youth group and decided my father was a sinful adulterer. Now I was the adulterer and for the first time in my life, I couldn't look my mother in the eyes.

Like the Haitian roads, these new feelings about her made me feel seasick and strange. Every time I saw her, I felt guilty for leaving Dick, for wounding him the way her husbands had wounded her. Dick and I had no children or property to bicker over. But that didn't mean I wasn't guilty. I slept with Rus the night before I left Dick and it wasn't love at the time, it was lust; it was just the kind of amoral behavior—adultery, the scarlet "A"—that I had self-righteously railed against since my parents' divorce. And the fact that I did it was what shocked me into finally moving out.

And just as Mom had not deserved to be tossed aside by two husbands, Dick didn't deserve to be tossed aside by me. On a good day, he was gentle and funny and his Carolina accent charmed me and everyone else. On a good night, he was long-limbed and surfer-blond and lazily sensual, just like when we met, two lucky, literature-loving American exchange students washed up on the shores of England in the dirt-cheap, Punk Rock seventies. But on most days and nights, he was un-gently, un-funnily depressed. He wanted to be a writer, but wasn't writing. He was teaching a few community college classes, but didn't like it much. He needed to get another job, but wasn't getting one. He liked Seattle, but the weather was killing him. I was the breadwinner, but my salary was about what a rookie schoolteacher would make. I was running out of patience and sympathy. I was tired of feeling guilty for liking my job and my hyperactive, creative, risk-loving work friends. I was tired of coming home to gloom. I was tired of trying to cheerlead.

I was tired of being tired. I was too young to be so tired. Rus made me feel like I would never ever feel tired again.

For months after that night, I felt like the new Bad Girl who'd never been bad before and didn't really know how to wear the label. The gossip at the TV station wasn't about Rus—after all, he was single, good-looking and arrogant—it was about me: married, serious, hard-working me, the one you went to when you needed help with your script or your research. Not the one you went to for a one-night stand. I was the producer who made the anchors look smart. I was not some ditzy airhead, some wannabe reporter. I was brainy. I'd gone back east to college. *How dare that Rus—with his one "s" and his python boots and his mustache and his show-offy, low-angle shots—how dare he break up her nice marriage to that cute teacher with the fetching Southern accent. What a jerk! Ann and Dick were our role models for young marriage! Now what will we do?*

The potholed road ground on and on. Rus cradled his camera. It was too dusty and bumpy to shoot much out the window.

As the crow flies, we couldn't have been far from the mountains of the D.R., where, three days earlier, we'd filmed volunteers helping local farmers plant trees in rich, black soil.

And then we rounded a sharp bend and found ourselves passing through a town right on the D.R. border, where, even though we were not leaving the country, Haitian soldiers, teenagers with machine guns, stopped us.

They asked for our passports. We handed them over. I looked around, trying to appear relaxed. There were just a few small buildings, tucked up against a grove of banana trees that had seen better days. A half-dozen bony dogs rested in the shade.

Rus nudged me and pointed with his eyes back to the soldiers. They were examining our passports upside down. Then they closed them and motioned us and our driver out of the car and into a dark, concrete hut that appeared to be a jail cell. They shut and locked the door, which in retrospect should have scared us more than it did. But it all happened so quickly and non-aggressively, as if they were simply short on space and the jail cell doubled as a waiting room, that it seemed logical to comply.

There were people squatting on the floor of the cell, eating mush from tin plates, looking like they'd been there a while. Through the bars of the door, we could see the soldiers showing our passports to another soldier sitting at a wooden table in the thin shade of the anemic banana trees. The prisoners, if they were prisoners, openly stared at us, but in a bored way, like this happened all the time.

Standing there with Rus, I felt detached from the scene around us, as if I knew I should be afraid, but it was all so sudden and surreal that I wasn't. And—and I knew this didn't make sense to people, so I didn't talk about it much—secretly, inside, I always felt so deeply good when I was with him that it cancelled out physical fear. I felt clean and honest. Baptized, in a way the teen youth minister might have understood. All my fakery had been washed away.

And something important was happening with Rus, something that might have a future. We were doing creative work together: long, atmosphere-drenched pieces that were more like short films than news stories. For many months now, we had been spending most of our free time with each other too, making a satirical movie just for fun with our friends, drinking beer at the Virginia Inn on First Avenue, eating after midnight at Tai Tung's or the 13 Coins, calling in to work in the morning to say we were at the "library" doing "research." We both lived in studio apartments, his in Wallingford and mine on Queen Anne Hill, and we shuttled back and forth across the Aurora Bridge from one to the other, blasting X in his car and Patsy Cline in mine. I had a better bed and a crow's-nest view of Lake Union; he had a VCR and the all-night Food Giant right next door.

We held hands and kept our faces neutral. We tried to project patience.

Then the officer at the table said a few words to the soldiers and handed our passports back. One of them unlocked the cell door, gave us our passports and waved us away.

Back in the car, I felt a little shaky.

I couldn't believe my mom was coming to this country. I couldn't believe Caroline was living here. Caroline was so young, and Mom was—not so young. And they didn't have the magical protection of love, like I did. The Fourth World, journalists had taken to calling Haiti, and I was beginning to understand why. If the green but poor D.R. was the third world, then this was a universe beyond: where dirt had gone to dust and green to brown and soldiers who couldn't read carried guns as big as themselves.

Looking back, there's something else I wonder: exactly when had I started worrying about Mom and whether or not she could handle a challenge?

One of my earliest memories is of our old pastel-green Pontiac sedan breaking down on a street in an unfamiliar neighborhood far from our own. It was just Mom and Lisa, then a baby, and me in the car. I don't know where we'd been. But I remember Mom scooping up Lisa and taking my hand and walking until we found a bus stop, all the while talking about what an adventure we were having: my first bus ride! In my three-year-old mind, it was the ideal moment: the complete safety of Mom, the thrilling adventure of the bus.

Our mother was the opposite of fear, the opposite of worry, the handler of everything. Two divorces didn't change that. Only when her third husband Ron died of cancer two months after they got married did it become conceivable to worry about her. But we never doubted that she would bounce back. And she did. Mostly.

Mostly. There were little things. But looking back, how to parse them? Women in their fifties love to blame forgetfulness on hormones: I know. Was Mom's fifty-something forgetfulness—a birthday here, a name there—just that, hormones, menopause, or was it something else? And what about the post-divorce pluckiness of her forties: had it become a little edgier, a little feistier, or were we imagining it? She seemed—defensive. As if something was nagging at her. Something she couldn't or wouldn't name.

At moments in my own life when it might have made more sense to babble in fear—like those moments in the Haitian border town jail—I often found myself mimicking her calm pluckiness. I knew I wasn't as brave as she was, but after watching her do it, I knew how to pretend. It was a great gift.

In 1987, it was still way too soon to believe that she might not be able to keep it up forever.

A few towns down the road from the border, we found Chris, the Peace Corps volunteer, in a hut with a woman whose leg had been badly burned in a cooking fire. Chris explained to us that she had treated the wound in the traditional Haitian way, basting it with bluing and raw egg, and it had become inflamed and possibly infected. He was soothing her in Kreyol and translating for a newly arrived doctor from Doctors Without Borders. Rus started shooting. I tried to keep the videotape deck—still cumbersomely attached by a long cable to the camera in those primitive video days—out of the dust. Chris had been in the Peace Corps for almost two years and it was clear that the woman with the burn knew him as a trusted friend, not one of the awkward outsiders the rest of us so clearly were.

Later, Chris took us to his favorite viewpoint, where he went when he needed to take a few deep breaths. Along the way, he talked about being a tall, red-headed, freckled Blanc, about standing out so much that eventually you don't stand out, you're just another quirk in the local landscape, like a tree that's been split in two by lightning. The fourth world.

The next day, we went to the Peace Corps' office in Port-au-Prince to meet Caroline. At first the office seemed empty, so I ducked into a bathroom while Rus waited. When I came out, I saw her over his shoulder, coming towards us down the dark hallway, the first time I'd seen her in seven months, her short braids swinging, her face lighting up at the sight of us. She looked like a younger, more wholesome version of myself. Part of me longed to be her: uncorrupted, idealistic, just starting out.

Rus told me later he saw Caroline before I came out of the bathroom and thought for a disoriented moment that she was me. He had not met her before. Both of us resembled our mom and all her tough Finnish ancestors: olive-skinned, blue-eyed, and strong-limbed. She and Mom had the same dark, straight hair. Mine was sandy. In a Bergman movie, we would be cast as the maids and cooks to the blonde stars.

What do sisters say when they haven't seen each other for a long

14

time? Nothing at first: you smile, laugh, embrace; in a split-second, you take in the changes—skin very brown and shiny in this heat, the female Peace Corps volunteer's de facto uniform of a modest top and loose skirt and running shoes—and you exult in the familiar: the sameness of the smile, the goofy little-girl laugh, the voice pitched, like Mom's, a good couple of octaves higher than my own. The no-nonsense hug of a youngest child who was over-held and over-hugged and treated like a new toy for four years by five older siblings, then suddenly dropped off a year early up at the Catholic school's all-day kindergarten when Mom and Dad got divorced and Mom became a full-time student and we big brothers and sisters became mini-parents mired in varying stages of adolescence.

"And of course this is Rus. And Rus, this is Caroline. I'm so happy you're finally meeting."

They did the awkward, first-meeting half-hug, all of us laughing to break the ice and then agreeing, yes, we'd better go get Mom at the airport.

I confessed to Caroline right away that I'd been brooding about Mom.

"Really?" she said. "Wow. That really surprises me. My Peace Corps friends are awed that Mom is visiting. Awed. They all have parents who are too worried about AIDS and the Tonton Macoutes to come visit and, you know, they don't like seeing poor people when they go to Mexico, so God knows they can't handle Haiti."

We followed her out of the office and across the narrow walkway that connected the ramshackle Peace Corps building, which was built out from the side of a steep hill, to the street.

"Besides," Caroline continued, "maybe this is hard for you to believe since you just turned THIRTY, but I'm still young enough to want a visit from Mom!" She clapped a platter-sized straw hat on her head.

"But I don't know if she's even thought about what she's getting into," I said, fumbling in my purse for my sunglasses. "She's been talking like it's going to be some big vacation, like the two of you are going to hang around a pool."

Caroline laughed. "Oh for God's sake, Ann, she's a teacher at a public high school in a big city. She has to face down 150 surly hormone cases a day. As she likes to say, she is a tough cookie! Is this your car? Nice!"

We waited while Rus fished out the keys.

"Speaking of cookies," Caroline continued, "I really hope she brought me some. I've been weirdly craving those Finnish Christmas ones with the chopped almonds, or Snickerdoodles, or even just some M&Ms . . . I told her anything that doesn't melt too fast would be great."

Rus listened with curiosity. He did not have much family. His parents split up after his only brother died at age nine during a botched operation to close a hole in his heart. Rus was seven at the time, with one older half-sister who was already out of the house. He grew up spending hours and hours alone. I grew up the third of six children, fantasizing about what it would be like to have privacy.

"We really should get going to the airport," he said, unlocking the doors.

"You sit in front and help Rus navigate." I climbed into the back seat. "Cookies. You *are* a dreamer. Didn't Mom have to get up in the middle of the night, Seattle time, to make her flight? And I think she had to turn in her quarter grades, I don't know, yesterday."

"She'll bring me something. I'm her baby, right?"

I reminded Caroline that Mom had grandchildren now. That the one thing she could count on her remembering to bring would be plenty of grandkid photos.

Caroline claimed she couldn't wait to hear all about our little niece and nephews.

"I know I must sound so cranky, Caroline," I said, as Rus inched out onto the main road. "It's just been weird with Mom lately. She doesn't listen. Or you think she's listening, but then she doesn't remember a thing." I tried to explain how odd it had been talking to Mom about Haiti, how she seemed only barely to compute that I would be there too. With Rus. For work. How it was as if I was talking about a trip that had nothing to do with hers.

"You'll tell her something important—like, guess what, Mom, the

16

news director says Rus and I can go to the D.R. and Haiti if we can get Pan Am to comp our airfare—and she'll say, 'Oh, great,' and then she'll just go off on some completely inane tangent about school or tennis or the grandkids."

Caroline was looking at me intently, her chin on the back of her seat, like I was speaking Kreyol or French and she was translating in her head as I talked.

"But that's how Mom is," she said. "She's always thinking about ten things at once."

"I know." Over Caroline's shoulder, I saw a man cross the street with a bird cage full of canaries balanced on his Panama hat. "But I guess I'm just worried she'll forget where she is, she'll forget to look out the window and see Haiti or ask you any questions about Haiti, because she'll be too busy talking about her flight or her last-minute packing or something."

I realized I couldn't even get near what was really bothering me: that Mom, through no fault of her own, made me feel like a bad girl instead of the joyously in-love girl I wanted to be every waking minute of the day—and I didn't know how to fix that. And I couldn't expect my youngest sister to fix it for me.

"You forget I've spent the last five summers living with Mom," Caroline said. "I'm used to her. It's going to be OK." She turned around. "Oh my God, Rus, turn here! Sorry!"

The man with the canaries danced to one side to avoid colliding with us and then danced again around a woman with a baby on one hip, her other arm reaching up to steady the dozen or so bolts of cloth piled high on her head.

I wanted to be in the present, in Haiti, with Caroline, with Rus. I wanted to see, hear, smell, taste the present. Mom was not the present.

We pulled up to the airport. Caroline and I went in and we spotted her right away, coming through the swinging doors, pushing her bags on a trolley. Right into the middle of my romantic fantasy. Right here, right now, in my treasured present, looking sweaty and a little bedraggled but in great spirits, like she'd been gardening all morning and just laid down

17

her tools for a lunch break. When she saw us, her knockout, I-love-you smile lit up her face and her arms opened and Caroline dove right into that hug, that hug I miss so much, these twenty-three years later, that I smell and feel it in my dreams.

One night, shortly after I left Dick, I was staying at my Dad's house while he and my stepmom were out of town and I started crying about what I'd done—how I'd ended something, *killed* something that had started so sweetly. I couldn't stop. Really couldn't stop. For hours. I finally called Mom. I don't know what time it was. I just know that she got out of bed, threw on some clothes, drove the two miles to Dad's and wrapped me in her hug and stroked my hair like I was still her little girl until, finally, I could stop. Even though I was a bad girl. Even though the next day and every day since, I still couldn't look her in the eye.

Rus took her bags and we headed to the car. Sure enough, she was full of stories about her flight: which friend gave her a ride to the airport; how hard it was to decide which and how many skirts and shirts to pack; how she was glad Caroline had advised us not to wear shorts, since she was feeling a little out of shape. She had M&Ms for all of us.

"Of course I brought lots of photos, too, but those can wait!" she said.

I watched out the window as we drove through what I now knew were the streets surrounding the Iron Market, Port-au-Prince's vast bazaar, where you could buy a cup of rice or a side of beef, a plastic bowl or a nesting set of ten, a giant wooden spoon, fruits that looked like stars. And peanuts, everywhere peanuts roasting over tiny fires.

At the Hotel Montana, the first thing Mom did was turn on the faucet and fill and drink a large glass of water before anyone could stop her.

"Mom, are you kidding? Did you really just do that? We're in Haiti!"

She looked at the glass like it had just appeared in her hand.

"Remember how I was telling you how careful you have to be? You can't drink the water here, not in this hotel, not anywhere!"

"Well, Ms. Smartypants, if I get sick I get sick!" She laughed and set the glass down. "Too late now!"

She did not get sick. Which was maddening, since I'd already flamed out gastro-intestinally speaking in the D.R., after being as careful as

I knew how, and Caroline's gut still wasn't behaving after six months in Haiti. Mom was indeed a tough cookie. Maybe it was her miner's daughter upbringing in Butte, Montana, her childhood spent drinking the water that bubbled up from under the copper deposits.

Caroline had drawn a luckier Peace Corps card than Chris, the volunteer we'd visited the day before. She was assigned to verdant Cap Rouge, perched on a cliff above the resort town of Jacmel on Haiti's southern coast. Because tourists went to Jacmel, there was a passable highway. The plan was to spend the night at the Stride Rite apartment, then set out the next morning in our rented Montero.

The next day, on the drive to Jacmel, we saw the Haiti that tourists and artists come to see: the sweeping red cliffs and valleys and distant views of the sea. There were no potholes; there were no teen soldiers. As we approached Jacmel, we saw vendors on the side of the road, selling oil paintings and gourds and soft drinks. Mom was charmed. She snapped photos. She paid attention as Caroline pointed out the cliff of Cap Rouge, where she lived in a house far too tiny to accommodate all of us and where we would go tomorrow for the day.

"It doesn't look far, but it'll take at least an hour," Caroline said. "The road is so steep you have to do it all in low gear. And you can't drive it, period, in the rainy season. But isn't it beautiful?"

We agreed that it was. And looking up at Cap Rouge, I was amazed that Caroline, barely twenty-two and fresh out of college, was doing this: living on a cliff in a Haitian village, one of two volunteers, the only two Blancs in the area. Speaking Kreyol with ease. Telling us about the preventive health care program she was helping to start. Such a very short time ago, I had been in college and she had been sending me color-crayoned pictures of our family and our house in Seattle. Then she'd become our token preppie, the only one of the six of us to go to a fancy private high school, and I'd worried she'd wind up with some Wall Street guy, living a Ralph Lauren kind of life. But no, here she was in her running shoes and peasant skirt, pointing out the sights in Haiti, talking to the roadside vendors in Kreyol.

It was Easter season and Jacmel was busy. Caroline had booked a room at a bed-and-breakfast in town for herself and Mom and a room at a hotel on a tiny cove outside of town for Rus and me. We dropped them off and doubled back to the Hotel Cyvadier.

If the Montana was the Sleeping Beauty Castle of Haiti's hotels, then the Cyvadier was like the funny fairy godmothers' quirky cottage. The manager, a French woman, was long-haired and plump and looked like she'd be comfortable mixing a potion or chanting a spell. Her one employee, the bellhop/waiter/bartender who took us to our bougainvillea-shaded room and brought us cold beers, insisted his name was "Je Veux."

"I want," he said. "Just say, 'Je Veux,' and I will be there."

"I want the beach," Rus said.

The path to the Cyvadier's beach was like a hand-made shore trail back home: first, the dirt track through a shady thicket, then the bleached, battered staircase, then the tangle of driftwood and rocks. But it was hot, beautifully hot, and the sand was as fine as sugar and the water silky and warm. We were the only Blancs in the cove. Down the beach, we could see some boys hammering and painting away on what looked to us like the wreckage of a boat. They waved cheerfully when they saw us and we waved back.

We both ran in, plunged under the waves and came up in the waist-high surf.

"Back in a minute," I said. "I can't resist."

Rus had not grown up swimming and he didn't like deep water, but I knew he liked to watch me swim. I dove under and swam hard out into the middle of the bay. It felt so good after days in jeeps and planes and cars, days of being dusty, sweaty, alert, polite. Now it was just us two in our own private cove. I flipped over on my back for a few minutes, letting the sun bake my face. Then I swam back towards Rus, dipping under water for the last few strokes and coming up right in front of him.

Standing in the lapping waves of the Cyvadier's cove, we kissed for a long time. And then Rus suddenly went all shy and awkward. He pulled back to look at me, keeping his hands on my waist. His sexy, deep-set, caramel eyes had a newly hesitant look. I thought he was getting

20

nervous about being in the water for so long. Or maybe he was bothered by the boys down the beach who were whistling and catcalling at us in a harmless, joking way.

But no, he was asking me to marry him. And I was saying yes.

"After all, only a fool would propose on April Fool's Day and not mean it," he said.

"Yes," I said. "Yes, yes, yes. Je veux."

Yes, je veux, even though I had no idea what it would mean or how it would all unfold. But at that moment in Haiti, there wasn't an iota of *No* or *Maybe* or *Let's think about it* in me.

We kissed some more and found ourselves laughing because it all felt so absurdly good.

We still had two hours until dinner and there were cold beers in a bucket in our room. As we peeled off our swimsuits, Rus told me he'd thought of proposing one night at the D.R., but was glad he'd waited, especially since I ate something bad that night and did a lot of throwing up. I tossed back the sheets and said thank God he hadn't on that night and the Cyvadier was perfect, being in this bed all salty and sandy and clinking our Prestige beer bottles was perfect. We would always remember this: saying yes, starting out together, in Haiti.

On the drive back into town to meet Mom and Caroline and Caroline's Peace Corps colleague Peter for dinner, I was brimming, full, flooded with love for Rus and Caroline and, yes, Mom and oh yeah, Peter, who I hadn't met yet, and all of humankind. It was April first. Rus and I had a whole future ahead of us. Everything was beautiful. Haiti was beautiful.

But twenty-three years later, I can see some of what I couldn't see at that moment on April Fool's Day, 1987. I can see my mother, a woman closer in age to me now than me then, so excited about trading in her everyday worries for the thrill of getting on a plane and flying to a part of the world she had never visited, where not one but two grown daughters would be waiting for her, two of her six children. Her children were now all college graduates, every one of them, and she would brag about it more if it just didn't sound so obnoxious. Six children launched! Four married, well, three now, and three grandchildren already. She'd been raising children since she was twenty years old and more than half that time, she'd been doing it alone. She deserved this trip and she intended to enjoy it. So what if she'd have to do some catching up on paper grading when she got home. So what if her penny-pinching ex-husbands disapproved. Think of what they missed by not taking trips like this to see their kids. And those nagging fears about her brain misfiring, about reaching for a word in front of the classroom and coming up blank: well, wouldn't a complete change of pace be just the thing?

And then there was Caroline. Floating along like I was on that blissful afternoon made me just as unable to fathom the tremendously daring cliff dive she had just made from college to Haiti. I thought I understood. But really I was just seeing her in relation to me and to Rus. I was proud to be showing them off to each other: my new boyfriend, the hotshot cameraman, and my cool little sister, the Peace Corps volunteer. I wasn't thinking about what it must have meant to her to have her mom and her big sister visiting her in this, her first seriously responsible gig as an adult, a gig she had barely begun and which she knew could turn out to be far more difficult and even dangerous than she had told any of us. And yet, because it meant I could come see her, she was allowing me to turn it into a TV news story, of all things. She would be showing us her world. She would no longer be the baby of the family. And she had promised herself she would be very mature about meeting the new boyfriend, even though she missed Dick.

We were gathering at the Hotel Jacmelienne, a white-pillared, aging doyenne of a place that seemed, in my awash-with-love mode, perfect for the occasion, even though, in the brief tropical twilight, its narrow, open-air bar was already as dark as a movie theatre just before the film begins.

Caroline introduced us to Peter, the only other Peace Corps volunteer in the Jacmel area, who had been there a little longer than she had. We sat down, our backs to the ocean, facing Mom, Peter, and Caroline across a tiny table, our eyes adjusting clumsily to the low light. Peter, skinny and blond, was only a few years older than Caroline and she had told us he was looking forward to a family kind of an evening, even if it wasn't his family.

And then I couldn't wait another minute.

"Well, I have some big news. Rus and I are engaged! As of about two hours ago!"

There were a few strange seconds of silence. Then exclamations and kisses from Mom, handshakes and congratulations from Peter.

And then Caroline began to cry.

Caroline, who'd whispered to me just that morning how much she liked Rus. Caroline, who I had counted on to be my ally if Mom flipped out about our engagement.

"I'm so, so sorry," she said. "I really am happy for you guys. It's just that—well you know I liked Dick too and it's weird to think he's just gone and—" She stopped and dabbed her eyes with her napkin and laughed a little in the middle of crying. "—And I really like you, Rus, I do, and I can see how happy you guys are, but I guess I need to get used to all this."

Seeing Caroline cry made me cry. We hugged and cried together. I don't remember what Rus and Peter did. But Mom took action.

"Well, I think what we need is some champagne!" she said, and she stood up and headed into the shadowy depths of the bar. "My treat. I insist."

"Caroline," I said. "I feel so incredibly stupid. I hadn't even thought about what this would be like for you. I am so sorry."

"No, really, it's OK. You can't exactly keep news like that to yourself, can you? It's just that feeling—when you're prepared for all kinds of stuff but not for the thing that actually happens, you know?"

Meanwhile, Rus was explaining to Peter about our history and my divorce and how Caroline had still been a kid when Dick and I got together, which I hadn't really thought about until I heard him say it.

Quite a few minutes later, Mom and a waiter returned with a dusty bottle of champagne and glasses. "To Ann and Rus," she toasted. "Long life and happiness and many children!"

We dried our tears and laughed and drank, and drank some more. I felt so happy that she was happy for us. Of course she wanted me to be in love. Of course she understood everything and didn't think I was awful. What a fool I'd been. What a self-centered idiot.

Warmed by the champagne, Caroline and Peter and Rus and I began to talk about Haiti, politics, the Peace Corps. The sky was utterly black now and we huddled around the one candle on our table. I told them about the soldiers who stopped us at the D.R. border. They told us about rumors of Duvalierists planning a coup and Tonton Macoutes still at large, but they chose their words carefully, explaining that it was important to say things like, "followers of the former leader," so that nothing would leap out of our English conversation and catch the attention of the people around us. I had never been anywhere as volatile as Haiti and, over champagne in a bar in a tourist town, it was exotic and exciting, not frightening.

When our food finally arrived—crispy fish and fried bananas and sweet potatoes—we all ate and talked at the same time. Except for Mom, who wasn't eating or talking much at all, and her face was outside the circle of candlelight.

Looking back on that night, I can imagine her feeling, at first, nothing but happy for Rus and me—with maybe a little wistfulness about Dick—happy to be in Haiti, happy to be with Caroline, happy to be drinking champagne. But I can also imagine that she must have begun to feel very tired. She had gone from school one day to Haiti the next. Maybe she'd had another one of those moments in front of the class, when Shakespeare or Faulkner, her old friends, eluded her and her students shifted in their seats and exchanged knowing looks with each other. Maybe she'd had a moment with Dad, with him wondering aloud how she could afford such a trip or whether Caroline needed that kind of coddling. Maybe her Northern brain and body were saturated, overloaded, with the heat and color and noises and smells of Haiti. Maybe she hadn't eaten enough before we started drinking. None of us had, but we were all younger and not so tired.

After a while she leaned in and tried to say something and someone, it could have been any one of us, corrected her.

"Please don't patronize me." Her voice was suddenly a little too teacher-loud.

"Mom—" Caroline began.

"Let me TALK. Please."

Suddenly we were all on high alert.

"We're listening," I said.

"I just wish I knew what you all were talking about." Her volume was still uncomfortably high. "I haven't had time to study up on Haiti. But no one's even given me a chance to ask a question!" She laughed a little but it didn't sound right.

"Mom," I said. "I'm sorry."

"Well, me too. I guess I'm just a little tired, and that's no crime, is it?"

"Of course not," Caroline said.

"I must seem pretty dull to all of you."

"Mom, what are you talking about?" I leaned in towards her, trying to keep my voice low, hoping she'd follow suit.

"I guess I'm talking about feeling . . . well, to be frank, feeling ignored!" That odd laugh again.

"Mom, we didn't mean to ignore you. Rus and I don't know anything about Haiti either and we figured we could learn a few things from Caroline and Peter."

"Fine. Don't let me stop you."

"Mom, c'mon," Caroline tried. "Mom, please, we don't think—"

"Maybe I'll just head back to the room," she said, standing up, looking at me. "I'm happy for you, honey, I really am. Maybe we can have a real conversation about your plans when we get back to Seattle."

My face went red-hot. Mom never talked to me this way. She sounded like some other mom, someone else's bitter, sarcastic mom. Not the mom I knew. I could feel heads turning, eyes on us.

"Arlene," Rus said. "I'm sorry, I—we—you're right, we were being rude. I'm really sorry. Let's sit down and finish our meal."

"Finish our meal! I hardly think so. You eat all you want. I'll wait outside." She grabbed her purse and headed out the door.

"Mom, please," Caroline called as she followed her out of the bar. "What are you doing?"

Rus and Peter stood up and started pulling out American dollars and piling them on the table.

Outside, Mom was standing unnaturally still and staring into the darkness, away from us. She looked exhausted. She looked older than I'd ever seen her look: older than her age, instead of younger. Her spine was as straight as it always was but her face sagged.

Peter said good-night, quickly.

She turned to him like she wasn't quite sure who he was. "Good night," she said. Then she turned back to the three of us.

"Mom—" I began.

"Don't. Don't say anything more, please. I'm just so damned tired. And I'm tired of being patronized. By all you young people who think you've got it all figured out!"

Rus was shepherding us down the street, towards Mom and Caroline's bed and breakfast. He looked bewildered and a little like he wanted to flee.

We stood outside their door and Mom continued to rant about being tired and being patronized and Caroline and I continued to plead. Finally, Mom began to sob. She let Caroline hold her. We watched as the tears helped her calm down and then Caroline slowly led her inside, motioning us to follow and wait outside the room.

A few minutes later, Caroline opened the door and told us that she and Mom would be OK, that it would be best if Rus and I left now and we met in the morning after breakfast, as planned, for the drive to Cap Rouge.

We couldn't say it out loud, but I knew Caroline and I were both thinking the same thing: we had never, ever, seen Mom like this. This was not the Woman of Steel we knew. This was not the generous, champagne-buying Mom we'd known two hours ago. Even after Ron died, when Caroline was only twelve, Mom kept it together, at least in front of the kids. And whatever it was that made her snap at the Jacmelienne, it seemed to be more than our political discussion. It was something else. Something about feeling left out, but not in the emotional way that the words "left out" usually imply.

It was as if her brain felt left out. Left behind. And in 1987, that was not a feeling she was used to.

Rus and I drove slowly back to the Cyvadier. The night was moonless, pitch black, and yet there were people walking all along the highway, carrying baskets on their heads, going home, we supposed, but where were their homes in this darkness? They blinked in the glare of our headlights. The children we saw were too sleepy to smile or wave. We didn't talk about Mom. We had to concentrate on watching for the turnoff to the Cyvadier.

What a relief it was, to finally get in bed and curl up in Rus's arms and hear him tell me everything would be OK. That my mom had just had a long, strange couple of days and she was wiped out. I was too tired to do anything but nod my head and believe him and gratefully fall asleep.

The next morning, we picked Mom and Caroline up and headed up to Cap Rouge. None of us said anything about the evening at the Jacmelienne. We talked instead about how dark it was at night but how early and quickly the sun rose, how good our breakfast coffee was, how truly red these cliffs were, what we hoped to film that day.

The town of Cap Rouge was a cluster of huts on either side of a dusty path not quite wide enough to call a road. It was market day. The vendors set their baskets on the ground along the central path. Caroline chatted with them, buying rice and beans and peanuts and bananas. Rus and I followed with the camera. Mom was busy taking pictures too and she was fine about not being part of our TV story, which we had all agreed would be too hard to explain to the news director. Later, we filmed Caroline meeting with the local people who would be her partners in the new health education program. Then we went back to her house and interviewed her at her tiny kitchen table.

In the afternoon, Caroline's neighbors came by to say hello. Everyone was so excited to meet us they could barely stand it. They were especially eager to meet Mom—imagine, the young Blanc Caroline's mother visiting all the way from Seattle, what an honor! Mom smiled and laughed, enjoying the attention, putting her arms around us and urging Caroline to tell everyone that Rus and I were engaged. The neighbors brought over extra chairs for us so we could eat our rice and beans sitting down.

It was a long day and a good day. We were all ready for bed by the time we drove back down to Jacmel.

The morning after that, Rus and I said good-bye and drove back to Port-au-Prince and flew home. Meanwhile, Caroline and Mom checked into the Cyvadier for a few days of R&R, which turned out not to be so restful: Mom slipped on the tile around the pool and had to limp through the rest of her trip.

Two decades later, I found a small bundle of Caroline's Peace Corps letters in a box in my closet.

One of them began, "Dear Ann, —Mom's last night."

"She and I had a good evening together, actually, Friday after you left," Caroline wrote. "She was talking about worrying about blanking out in front of her class on very common words. And her behavior over drinks at the Jacmelienne worried her too, she said. It freaked her out. I told her I was relieved to hear her say that because I was concerned too and worried that she seemed to dismiss it so easily. She said she was just embarrassed and didn't know how to bring it up. I was indeed relieved."

One of the very worst things about Alzheimer's disease is that you really don't know when it starts, let alone how or why. And of course we still don't with Mom. But I had long forgotten getting that letter. And Caroline had forgotten writing it.

We didn't remember it because in 1987, our mom was still what we thought of as herself: youthful, intrepid, willing to jump on a plane to Haiti. Not so good about remembering the details of our lives, but always so proud of us. Of course we could not erase the bad night in Jacmel. But for Rus and me, the afternoon of that day, saying *Yes* and *Je veux* at the Cyvadier, was such a sublime and defining moment of our lives that we couldn't dwell on what went wrong that evening. The story to tell when we got home was that we were engaged: crazy, but true!

Alzheimer's disease was the last thing on our minds.

Now, I stare at that line—"blanking out in front of the class on very common words"—and I am stunned to think that it started that long ago. Back when I was so selfish that all I could see, when I saw Mom, was the person who, without even trying, was making me feel guilty when all I wanted to feel was in love.

In Haiti, unbeknownst to us, Mom was walking into her own fourth world. A place where no amount of intervention could save her. An eroding landscape that would, in less than twenty years, scrub her dry.

Tonight, Tonight

"Please do me a favor," Mom asked me.

How often I've wondered what it was like to be her. To struggle to think, the way people with pneumonia struggle to breathe.

"OK, a favor. I'll try," I said, squinting as the low sun flared.

It was December 2001. After two years at the Lakeview Retirement Community, we had just moved her to the Fairview Terrace, a new facility that specialized in Alzheimer's care. Mom and I were standing in a square of winter sun in her new snowy-white living space: one room with one window, one twin bed, one dresser and one chair. Her hair was fluffy-clean and haloed in the slanting light with flyaways, like a baby's; her clothes were unspotted. She looked better than she had in weeks. But her eyes were sheepish and pleading; they were the eyes of a little girl trying to charm her way out of big trouble.

She took a breath, and blurted, "Please—don't tell my family about this."

What she said made perfect sense—to her. In that moment, in her pleading eyes, I was not me, Ann, her third child, her firstborn of her second marriage, the mother of two of her fourteen grandkids. I was a stranger, sternly telling her that she was in trouble, that the woman she'd pushed out of bed the night before had required stitches and her family was livid and there would be consequences.

I hesitated, as I had taught myself to do with Mom, taking the two seconds I needed to make the decision. *Go along with this one. Just for the moment. She's overwhelmed. Don't take it personally.*

31

"OK," I said in a formal, I'm-a-stranger voice, and then, "Let's sit down for a minute."

But I wasn't a stranger. I was her daughter. And this was the first time she had ever done this: talked to me as if she didn't know me. It stunned me, it stung, the way it stings when someone you love tells you they don't love you anymore.

"I don't know what happened," she said. "I can't remember."

"I know, Mom. I know."

We sat down on the bed and I put my arm around her and that triggered something, because I could tell from the way her shoulder nested into me that I was her daughter again.

"It's that damned—thing I've got, that—"

"Alzheimer's."

"Yes. Alzheimer's."

Before our daughter was born, one of the gifts we received was a baby bath, featuring a baby-shaped, baby-sized sponge cushion that fit neatly into the white plastic bathtub. What a brilliant idea, I remember thinking. Our baby won't have to slip and slide on hard plastic; she or he (we still didn't know) will recline on this nice yellow sponge and gurgle with bath-time joy.

But after spending our first night at home with Claire, not sleeping more than five minutes at a time because we felt compelled to watch her, terrified, to make sure she kept breathing, Rus and I looked at the baby bath in the morning as if it were a complicated machine that we had no idea how to operate and we both had the same thought: call Arlene.

Like many pregnant women, I had vowed that I would declare my independence as a mother, not let my mom take over, I would do it my way. But that was before twenty hours of labor and three nights without sleep. My brain felt like used cheesecloth. It was hard enough to figure out breast feeding, let alone baby bathing. I needed Mom: her wisdom, her experience, her well-rested brain.

In the video Rus shot of Claire's first bath, Mom is smiling and chattering and holding eight pounds of wet, squalling newborn Claire with one hand while she turns on the kitchen faucet and checks the water temperature with the other. Claire is hollering loudly through the whole experience, but as soon as it's over, Mom wraps her in her hooded baby towel and holds her up to her shoulder, soothing her, cooing to her, and in seconds Claire is resting calmly in her arms, staring at me and Rus with a look that says, "Why can't you be more like her?" In the background, you can see me lurking like a zombie in my pink robe and huge glasses, looking like a just-risen pan of cinnamon rolls, puffy and doughy and dark-circled.

Now, Mom and I are sitting side by side on a twin bed in a room barely bigger than that tiny apartment kitchen. Claire is twelve. She has a little brother, Nick. They have happy memories of nights at Grandma's house, always eating exactly the same meal—Mom's chewy beef stew, with Rocky Road ice cream for dessert—and watching the same movie—*West Side Story*, always ejected before the bloodshed starts. But those overnights ended a long time ago. Now, Mom's life has shrunk to one room. She can't keep her own stash of ice cream anymore, or watch her own movies on her own TV.

A healthy brain resembles a big, expensive sponge from a fancy bath store, plump and absorbent and ready to cleanse you in a constant, rejuvenating waterfall of new thoughts, emotions, reflexes, actions, prayers, insights. A brain afflicted with Alzheimer's disease gradually starts to look like the old, smelly, dried-up sponge that you keep trying to use until you come to your senses and demote it from the kitchen sink to the basement sink, where you leave it to shrivel for months before someone finally throws it away. You can't do much with a sponge like that. It's stiff and dry and water runs right off of it.

During the *West Side Story* years, Claire would come home after a night at Grandma's, put on what she called her Maria nightgown, pull the step stool from the kitchen into the middle of the living room, climb up the two steps and sing down to Tony from her fire escape. "Tonight, tonight," she would serenade with feeling, "won't be just any night. Tonight there will be no morning star . . ."

When I was a little girl, Mom belted out "Tonight" and "I Feel Pretty" while she did the laundry, which was often. There were eight of us. There were mountains of diapers and sheets and T-shirts and tights and my brother's football gear and Dad's tennis whites. Mom had never been to New York in her life. But the songs lifted her out of our dank, laundry-filled Seattle basement and onto the fire escapes of Manhattan, where romance and hope blossomed briefly. "Oh moon, go bright, and make this endless day endless night . . ."

What Claire and I learned from Mom and *West Side Story* was this: Don't let the piles of laundry stop you. There is passion waiting on the fire escape and in the back of the dress shop and on the rooftops and at the dance in the gym. If you're stuck, for now, with the laundry, or with a step stool in your living room, then let your imagination take you there.

And so I have to wonder, because someday I could be Mom: where does your imagination take you when plaques and tangles are blocking the way?

Someday I could be Mom, that's a place I try not to go too often, not on purpose. I tell myself that it could have been all those toxins in Butte, Montana that triggered Alzheimer's disease in Mom, or maybe a combination of toxins and stress: losing two husbands to divorce and one to death. I remind myself that we don't have a strong family history of Alzheimer's. But the fear is always there, always, and it was there even before we knew that what was wrong with Mom was Alzheimer's, back when Claire and Nick were toddlers and we thought maybe she was still distracted by grief over the death of Ron, her third husband, or maybe she was just plain lonely, even though she claimed to be loving her empty nest.

Back then, what I feared was that someday I would allow my life to become what Mom was allowing hers to become: a life of puttering.

"What'd you do today, Mom?" I'd ask.

"Oh, nothing much. Just puttered around."

Puttering meant a little cleaning, a little weeding, a little laundry; it meant the crossword, *Time* magazine, TV shows she'd never previously had time to watch, like *Columbo*. She loved Peter Falk in his rumpled raincoat. No harm in all that. She had quit teaching the year Nick was born, a year before her scheduled retirement, because those blank-outs in front of the class that began some time before she went to Haiti had started happening so often that she'd lost her confidence. Don't be so judgmental, I would scold myself. Nothing wrong with taking it easy after all those years in the classroom. But she wasn't reading books. She was painting less and less. She said she wanted to write her story, but her boxy new Mac was gathering dust. All she did was putter.

What drama there was in her life was caused by her own distraction: She would forget to grab a house key when she went out for a walk and find herself locked out, again. She would forget where she parked the car when she went downtown to shop and it would be towed. Again.

It was exactly during the years when I was busy trying to figure out how to juggle being a mother with being some kind of working creative person that Mom, the former powerhouse of working motherhood, began to change before my eyes into a distracted putterer. I didn't want to think too hard about why this was happening. My days were full, so I had the convenient excuse of little time to dwell on how Mom was changing. And the circular sameness of her activities actually made her a great refuge for my young children: she wasn't about to try anything ambitious or new; she was going to make beef stew and then curl up with them and watch *West Side Story*, but not the sad part.

And if I did start dwelling too much on how she was changing, I might have to say something and that would just open a can of worms: "Mom, I think you're depressed." "Mom, have you considered volunteering?"

I actually tried that line once and she looked at me like I was nuts. "I spent all those years teaching and now you think I should volunteer?"

Before Mom's Alzheimer's had a name, what I feared when I looked at her life was loneliness and lack of purpose. If I wind up alone like Mom, I would vow, I will work, I will write, I will volunteer, I will make sure my life has meaning.

After we learned that she had Alzheimer's disease and that she'd probably had it for years, I was ashamed of the way I had judged her so arrogantly, especially as the small indignities started to pile up: She was dropped from the tennis roster at the Tennis Club. She was dropped from her bridge group. On her last trip to Europe, she had decided to take a walk while the rest of her tour group was resting and she got lost in Lisbon and could not remember the name of her hotel. She walked into another hotel and a good-hearted desk clerk helped her figure it out and put her in a taxi, but for her it was a new low, an embarrassing turning point.

Back then, I was too busy trying to make her feel better to dwell on how awful it must have been. Now, I can dwell all I want.

I can picture her in her tennis outfit, sitting at the table in her bright yellow kitchen with its heart-stopping view of Mount Rainier, calling the club on a Tuesday morning to get her Ladies' Day tennis time.

"Sorry, Arlene, you're not on the list."

And then what did they say?

Was it, "We've had complaints that you can't stay in the game anymore"? or, "We hear you've been diagnosed and well, we know where that's going"?

After years of blaming the Tennis Club for all kinds of things, from my own social awkwardness to actually causing my parents' divorce, now I had a whole new grievance to add to the list. But is that fair? What do you do when someone who is physically fit but whose brain is shot still wants to play tennis?

I picture Mom hanging up the phone and staring out at the mountain and the water and trying to take this in: she has just been fired from playing tennis, a sport she has enjoyed for forty years.

Maybe she got up and watered the plants or folded some laundry.

Maybe I called to remind her that she had offered to babysit that night, so she got some stew meat out of the freezer and checked to make sure she had ice cream.

Maybe I asked her if she was looking forward to playing tennis on such a nice day and she said, "Oh, I'm not going to play, my shoulder's bothering me."

And I probably thought, Wow, now she's even cutting out tennis. This Alzheimer's diagnosis really has her down. If only I could get her to volunteer at the kids' school.

What an idiot I was. What did I know about Alzheimer's? About getting through the days never knowing when your brain might hit a roadblock, never knowing when you might be newly humiliated?

The tennis ball's coming her way and she knows she's supposed to raise her racket and return it but she—doesn't. The message doesn't get from her clogged-up brain down to her arm fast enough.

Key, *she says a dozen times,* Grab the key on your way out the door. *But then the door closes behind her, locked tight, and she realizes the key is still sitting on the table, right inside.*

Pine Street. Eighth and Pine. Picture the eight. Picture a pine tree. That's where the car is. *But after an hour of shopping, she can't picture the car anywhere at all. She can't even remember what kind of car she drives.*

"You're so lucky, Arlene," her friends would say. "You have so many children to help you out when you need it."

But her friends didn't know what it was like to call her busy daughter, who was doing some kind of freelancing but she could never remember what, and her daughter might be at home but she might not. They didn't know what it was like to have to say, "I lost the car. Again." Or "I'm locked out. Again." They didn't know what it was like to feel ashamed around her own children.

And, though she didn't want to imagine it, she did know, with some part of the brain she still had, she did know that it was going to get worse. And then keep on getting worse. Tonight there will be no morning star. At least her friends who had, say, cancer could let their imaginations take them to a place where they might be cured.

Instead of to a single room with a single bed, where she has to sit and listen while her daughter tells her what a bad, bad thing she's done. A thing she can't even remember doing. And now there would be consequences? What consequences?

37

"Why is there something instead of nothing?" The *New York Times* asked one day in an editorial. Why a universe, instead of oblivion? Why life? The *Times* wrote that physicists have concluded that "it all comes down to a very slight bias, an asymmetry, in the behavior of a subatomic particle, the neutral B-meson. As it oscillates between its matter and antimatter states, it shows a slight predilection for matter."

A very slight bias. An asymmetry, oscillating towards matter. As the stardust that was my mother met the stardust that is my father, they edged toward creating something instead of nothing. A marriage. A family. A whole chain of somethings: My sisters and brothers and me. Our relationships. Our children. Lives and lives and lives.

And like every human before me, I wonder: what if there had been nothing instead of the something that became us? The flawed, messy, loving something that was us. The *something* whose beating heart was Mom.

I was very young when I started wondering too much. Sometimes my brain just floated away from the joys of matter—toes in sand, tongue on soft-serve ice cream—to the gaping void of antimatter. It terrified me. When I was in kindergarten, there were days when my head hurt from thinking. There were times when I strained so hard when I was thinking that I started crying. It happened one September night when the setting sun blazed up in the kitchen window as orange as a campfire and everything inside, including me, including Mom, was suddenly as dark as shadow puppets. She and I were putting dishes in the dishwasher—I was lining up the milk glasses, Flintstone glasses from the gas station—and the sun shot an orange beam right through them, right through Fred and Wilma and Pebbles and I burst into tears and said, "Oh, Mommy, I don't ever want to die!" and she said, "Oh, Annie," and wrapped me in a big hug and I wanted her to say more but at least she gave my hurting head a place to rest for a few minutes. A place to close my eyes until the orange went away.

This is how I remember Mom from the earliest years of my life: always, firmly, pulling me back from darkness, back to the lovely, light-filled asymmetry of the day. Back to putting the glasses in the dishwasher or stretching with Jack LaLanne or watching her iron Dad's shirts, the hot, heavenly starch scent filling the house. Mom's bias towards something versus nothing was inviolable. In her world, everything was good and nothing was perfect, and she liked to make a point of that: of the joy that comes with accepting asymmetry, unpredictability, spills, bruises. She thought perfectionist housekeeping was sad and silly. She refused to read women's magazines. Her reading time was too precious and she still had a lot of classics to get through. Naptime was a sacred island of quiet: if you had graduated from actually napping, you sat quietly with your own book while Mom read hers.

From the chaos of a failed first marriage and the surprise of a sudden second marriage, she created a *something* that she encouraged us to feel was different than other families' *somethings:* we were a bit of a patch job, but weren't we lucky to be who we were?

I don't think she planned to be Different with a capital "D." I think she embraced it as the best strategy under the circumstances: being divorced in the mid-1950s marked her, as did moving into Laurelhurst, my childhood neighborhood, where most moms had been sorority girls at the University of Washington and many had even been society girls, actual debutantes—certainly not miners' daughters from oddball places like Butte, Montana. They set their hair on huge rollers; they wore girdles and skirts and pink lipstick. Mom got a pixie cut and wore black slacks. Our little brick house was on the modest, downhill side of Laurelhurst Playfield. It resembled the seven dwarves' cottage and was just as crowded. It was by far the most luxurious place my mother had ever lived.

And yet she exuded confidence. Not hubristically or loudly, but matter-of-factly. As if there was simply no reason not to.

We woke up in the morning knowing that she would be in the kitchen, pouring juice into six plastic glasses, ready for each one of us with a hug and a smile: not an inane, fake, Stepford-smile, but a real one, the kind that says, Call me nuts but I love being your mom. And yours and yours and yours. I love all six of you, I will never play favorites and you will never lack for breakfast, lunch, dinner, hugs and kisses.

Whatever worries she had about stretching the family budget she carried lightly, at least in front of us. Whatever other mysterious grownup stresses she felt—about cars or plumbing or the constant clashes between Dad and my big brother Johnny—she treated as annoyances that had to be dealt with: pesky, minor, not at all what really mattered.

What really mattered was making sure the youngest of us got a song and a story at bedtime. Weekly trips to the library. After-school graham crackers and milk. Clean piles of laundry, to be folded not by her but by us according to our weekly "jobs" schedule (never chores, she disliked the word *chores*).

And what mattered most of all was sitting down to dinner together. If you'd pressed me, at ten, I would have said that dinner at our house is noisy and happy and yeah, we bicker but we also have these indescribably silly moments and surprising moments and I don't know why but it's not like that at a lot of my friends' houses. I don't know why, but we're different.

It certainly had nothing to do with the food. Mom's meals were anything but astonishing. The mania for Julia Child passed her right by. She had six children and a hungry young husband and her repertoire was all about filling us up with foods from each of the four groups. She came up with combos she liked and she stuck to them: chicken went with biscuits and frozen peas, hamburgers with canned peaches and cottage cheese.

Dinnertime was chaotic—there were battles over the last biscuit; there were dramas over hated vegetables—and there was always talk, talk, talk. Family news, school news, news of the day—we skated through it quickly, colloquially, the dense layers deftly covered in a constantly evolving family shorthand. There was the week spent debating what to name Caroline, who had arrived a few weeks early and who we were calling "Baby" until we made up our minds. There was Johnny telling us about the colleges he wanted to go to: I remember thinking, *There's a college named* Harvey Mudd? There was teenaged Kristie explaining her clothing chart, which made it possible for her never to repeat the same outfit in any three-week period. There was Dad announcing that Lisa and I were now old enough to ski and would be coming along on the next trip. And, always, there was Mom, the calm conductor, moving us along when one topic got too heated, paying attention to who was and was not eating their broccoli, decreeing who would get the last drumstick.

I know that she marveled at this *something* she and Dad had created. That she took pride in not allowing herself to pine for what other somethings—college, career—she may have given up. It's easy, now, to look back and say, Aha! Surely it could not have been good for her brain to ban all pining, to repress so much!

But Mom was like that subatomic particle, always oscillating towards matter. Towards what *was*: her children, her husband, the laundry, what to cook for dinner. To oscillate the other way, to ever favor nothing over her own something, was unthinkable.

As unthinkable as a disease whose modus operandi is just that: to smother all the somethings that fill our brains, that make us who we are. To smother them right back to nothing. Matter to antimatter. Asymmetry to oblivion.

I feel pretty, oh so pretty, that the city should give me its key . . . I think I was ten when I finally got to see *West Side Story* on the screen. It is one of the movies that made me want to make movies, although I did not know that the first time I saw it. I had listened to the record all my life, knew all the words to all the songs, loved to stand at the top of the laundry chute and listen to Mom sing them, her voice ringing in the concrete basement: *See the pretty girl in that mirror, there!*

I know I saw it before I was eleven because eleven was the year I stopped being a little kid: my parents began their long and ugly break up, Martin Luther King and Bobby Kennedy were killed, my older brother Johnny was starting to yell a lot at the dinner table about the Vietnam War and the draft and what he would do if he drew a low number. But the night I saw *West Side Story* was before all of that. I was still just a girl who was thrilled to be going to the movies with my mom and big sister, especially, finally, to see *West Side Story,* the movie I knew Mom loved more than any other.

41

I was electrified by the opening aerial sweep into New York, by the brilliant purples and reds of the dance in the gym, by Tony singing "Something's Coming." And then—I was undone, devastated, overwhelmed by his death. I hated death because I couldn't grasp it, I couldn't understand it, it made no sense, especially when two people were in love the way Tony and Maria were in love—surely theirs was the kind of love that would triumph over death, not be destroyed by it. Watching my mom and big sister cry and cry, as Maria picked up the gun and shouted to the Jets and the Sharks gathered around her, gangsters who were really just kids, just pencil-legged teens like Johnny—"Did you leave a bullet for me, Chino?"—I couldn't believe anything could ever be so sad. I almost wished I hadn't seen it. But this was long before VCRs. You didn't take your kids to the movies and then leave before the tragic part.

I remember feeling so old. Not in a proud way, like I'm really growing up now—more like, I'm ten but I feel like I'm a hundred. Now I know, I thought, now I know what getting old is: It's knowing stuff you wish you didn't know. It's knowing that love is not just happy; it's horrible. It's knowing what tragedy is.

The grinding tragedy of Alzheimer's is that the horrible part of the movie can last a dozen years, or more. And you can't turn it off. Not in the physical sense: there is no Death with Dignity option for people with Alzheimer's, because they can't fully participate in such a decision, even if you live in a place where it might be actually legal. And of course there's no clear line—whoa, here comes the awful part, eject that tape. Because how do you measure quality of life? Does a single moment—tasting chocolate, for example, long after you remember the word "chocolate," long after you could independently get a square of it into your own mouth—does that moment of pleasure on your tongue mean you can still experience "quality of life"? Does responding to touch, warm skin on warm skin, mean you're remembering love?

What I loved about *West Side Story* and what I grew to love about making documentaries is that good movies use all the tools of all the arts: Music, color, line, composition. Dance and movement. Words, sung and spoken. When we were making *Quick Brown Fox*, our film about Mom and Alzheimer's, we found some very old strips of Super-8 that my grandfather had shot. One was from Mom's tenth birthday in 1941. She smiles and then leans in and blows out the candles on her cake. Other reels were dated from when Mom was in her early twenties and my older brother and sister were babies. Rus put this film in a little hand-crank viewer. He surrounded the viewer with photos, set up his tripod, and filmed this tableau while he cranked the viewer. Then he used some music from an old music box that played a sort of mournful organ tune, and he edited the segment to some narration that I wrote:

I woke up one recent morning thinking about Mom and Butte and her life and her Alzheimer's disease and how our lives really are like our own personal movies that we play, rewind, edit, watch without ceasing. But life is not quite the right word. Consciousness, maybe, or soul or self—our sense of who we are—that's the movie. Which means our neurons are the actual film stock, the raw material on which the movie that is each one of us is recorded in our brain. So what happens when the film is damaged? Or the projector starts gobbling it up? What happens if that was the one and only print?

Endless night, is that what happens?

I still don't understand death. I do pray; I do believe, most days, that there's a God; and I long to believe that we don't all just end in endless night. That there is more to who we are than our bodies or our brains.

In the end, Mom's brain was as useless as an old sponge. But I can't bear to think that her soul, her self, had already been thrown away.

The Tennis Club

There are women who just can't help the fact that they make men weak in the knees. There are women who have this power whether or not they have a bad head cold or a large pimple on their nose or a baby spit-up stain on their shoulder. I am not one of those women. When I was younger, this truth felt unfair, a shameful disability, a life-altering sorrow. But over the decades, I've learned, albeit reluctantly, the upside of invisibility, of blending in, of being Doris Day instead of Marilyn Monroe, middle-sized, of middle coloring, and for many years now, middle-aged. If a man does listen to me, I know it's because he's actually interested in what I'm saying. If a man does find me beautiful, I know it's a personal, real feeling about the real me, and not a sort of objectified Barbie doll kind of appreciation. And I love feeling beautiful, oh I love it, the way a woman who is beautiful every minute of every day probably can't even imagine. Once, years ago, I listened to a former model describe how hard it was to again and again be appreciated only ornamentally, and at the time, I thought I felt no sympathy at all—yet here I am, years later, still remembering that conversation, still marveling at what a different sort of burden that would be.

And of course I know it's not about looks, not completely. It's that whole mysterious business of confidence, the kind that is supposed to grow as you grow, as it has been so filmily described in hundreds of seventh grade "Now You're a Woman" filmstrips. My confidence just didn't kick in at all until I was about twenty and, like a malnourished infant, it never really grew properly.

Which is maybe not an entirely accurate way to describe what happened, because as a baby and as a little girl, I was well-nourished, confidence-wise, by that first and most important romantic figure in a girl's life: Dad. He swooped me up and twirled me around; he dabbed shaving cream on my nose and sang a silly song about Annabelle Brown. He loved my funny, deep voice. My malapropisms became part of his vocabulary: Mazagine. Yew Nork. Unicle Brunce instead of Uncle Bruce. He spent a whole summer standing in a pool, his fair skin frying, moving further and further from the edge, coaxing me until I could swim all the way across.

It was sometime between that summer and the seventh-grade filmstrip that I started to starve. Grownups were so bad at divorce back then. No one knew what to say or do and so they counseled each other to say little, especially to the children. I get that now. I no longer blame my dad for leaving in exactly the same year that I got a mouthful of braces, a stretchy training bra that came in a box and a terribly wrong pair of glasses, pointy when everyone else had just switched to ovals or hexagons. I no longer blame him for teaching me, without really meaning to, that I was now invisible. For not even trying to explain to his children that we shouldn't listen to what people said; he wasn't really trading Mom in for a woman who was a few years younger and played better tennis, much as it might look that way. I was a terrible tennis player. I was now the oldest of his three daughters, gone from funny and cute to mute and awkward in what felt like a few weeks. Where did that leave me?

A more confident girl, a more beautiful girl, might have put up a fight. Waged a campaign to stay visible. But—encumbered now with the glasses and the braces—I was sure I didn't stand a chance. My dad had made it clear what he wanted. He had cast his vote for the Tennis Club world, a world of suntanned women in white tennis dresses, a world of jewel-toned lipstick and jangling bracelets and jingling ice cubes in glasses full of gold: iced tea at three, Chablis at six, bourbon at seven. It was a pretty world. Up until the divorce, I enjoyed visiting it. There was a time when it had even seemed welcoming, reassuring in its routine: the long summer days that started with swim team in the morning and sometimes included the tension of a dreaded tennis lesson but then at last unspooled into the lazy afternoon salvation of the lake and the beach and soft-serve ice cream cones.

It was the summer of 1969 when my mother gave up chauffeuring us across town to the Tennis Club. She was a student now. No more packing the six of us and our hand-me-down swim team suits and our stained tennis shorts and our sorry wooden tennis rackets into the station wagon. Now, she waved goodbye in the morning and bicycled up the hill to the University of Washington campus. Kristie and Johnny were teenagers with summer jobs. That left twelve-year-old me in charge: of Lisa, nearly ten; James, almost six; and Caroline, who had just turned four. Most mornings, I let them watch cartoons in their pajamas, eating Cap'n Crunch out of the box, and then tried to make up for it by playing school or pioneers or walking everyone down the hill to the drugstore for candy or up the hill to the swing set in the park.

In the evenings, I read and re-read *Cheaper by the Dozen* and *Mr. Popper's Penguins* and *The Family Nobody Wanted*, a book about a mom and a dad who loved being parents so much that they just kept adopting more children. I rode my bike as far as I dared and came home as late as I dared. I wrote poems in secret steno notebooks.

A year ago, I went on a search mission through the boxes in our basement and found those notebooks. I put them in a bin and brought them up two flights of stairs and set them on a shelf near my desk. I peeked inside and caught a few words—*candles flickering, cathedral woods, a daisy growing in a sidewalk crack*—but I couldn't quite allow myself to keep reading. Later, I thought.

Later finally came along last week.

It's research, I told myself. I'm trying to write about Mom and Dad and their marriage and divorce because it's part of Mom's story, the story of her life, the story of the pile-up of stress that may or may not have been part of the deadly mix that triggered her Alzheimer's disease. I need to remember what it was like, those summers of being twelve and thirteen, when she was racing through college and I was babysitting and we were all getting used to a new kind of summer, a season that now featured much less of the Tennis Club and many more daisies in sidewalks.

But the act of remembering is hard to direct. And sometimes props—dusty steno notebooks for example—just get in the way.

What I truly, viscerally remember from that time is my face feeling perpetually hot. Especially if I try to recall any scene starring my dad. Before the details swim into focus, what I first remember is that warm pooling of blood somewhere behind my eyes, in my brain, in my ears, and how I hated the divorce for making me hate, like Maria at the end of *West Side Story* when she turns to the Sharks and the Jets, Tony's body lying between them, and shouts, "You have taught me to hate! You and you and you!"

This is what I remember. But there is nothing of this in the penciled poems that fill the spiral notebooks that I have saved for four decades. Nothing.

"We scooped the clouds with silver spoons," begins one poem.

"If I have no food, I will eat sunshine," begins another.

"A poem is a daydream on paper."

They're all like that, until they start getting religious.

"A Christian is an eternal fire."

"Thank you God/for letting me in/even though/I'll probably/get mud/on/your carpet."

I didn't write one word about Mom or Dad or the divorce. It's all clouds and sunsets and ladybugs and God. There are a few furtive poems about feeling lonely. And sometimes I wrote anti-war poems—"Waiting for that deadly cry,/waiting for the word/That tears him from his home . . ." But I wrote nothing, nothing at all, about the hate and sorrow that had ripped through my heart and head, that I tried to drown out by praying and writing poems about nature and focusing as hard as ever I could on goodness and light.

And what I remember is that it didn't work very well. Viscerally speaking.

It was 1969 and there was darkness not just in my heart but everywhere I looked: riots, war, hypocrisy. It was 1969 and I was twelve and everyone in the world was angry and my father was gone, living in a cramped apartment and spending his time with some other children and their mother. My big brother and sister had changed too: they weren't home much but when they were, they closed their doors and stayed in their rooms or they took over the living room stereo and played their music louder than ever. Meanwhile, my mother had left me to babysit while she tried to paper over her own broken heart with pages and pages of literature: Beowulf, Chaucer, Shakespeare, Dickens. And I didn't know how to write about all this darkness so I comforted myself by writing poems full of light.

The only people willing to acknowledge that the shape of the world was shifting and we all might need some help finding firm ground were the new youth group leaders at the church up the street, a church my parents had required my brothers and sisters and me to attend so that we would be "exposed" to religion, as if it were chicken pox and they wanted us to contract a mild childhood case in exchange for lifetime immunity. But I began going beyond exposure. I began paying attention. I wanted to hear them explain what life was supposed to mean. I needed to know, because it was clear to me that my parents did not know. I was so thirsty for what they had to say.

Even now, though I'm back in church in a grateful, muddled, middle-aged way, even now I wince when I remember my fervent adolescent faith: when I pick up the dog-eared Bible I bought at thirteen and underlined with yellow, pink, and aqua pens; when I find the old poems or leaf through my teenage journal, full of prayers and Lenten resolutions. I wince and I also wonder, because I've lost this specific bit of memory: I wonder at what moment, somewhere around age twelve, I began to really truly believe. Another question left unanswered by the scribble-filled steno books.

But last week, when I sat down to re-read the poems, I began to finally get past wincing and to marvel at what I had done.

What I thought I was—the apple of my father's eye—had just been ripped away from me. Where I thought I was—in the middle of a big family that spent its long summer days at a fancy club where everyone was richer than we were but hey, we didn't mind too much because we had each other—that was gone too. Who I was—a dreamy, nearsighted girl who could swim but couldn't play tennis, who liked knowing there was a book in her beach bag—that girl was gone.

Now I was a twelve-year-old who had responsibilities. And nowhere to swim.

Everything had changed, and there was this dangerous river of darkness running through the world and through me. But there was also a shore of sudden freedom. And I found it.

I found the freedom, suddenly, to decide all kinds of things. I decided to go to youth group and listen to what they had to say. No one made me go and no one stopped me. I decided to get up in the morning and watch the sun rise and write a poem about it. I decided a daisy in the crack of a sidewalk was worth describing. I may have had pointy, awful glasses but I also had my own brand-new form of 20/20 vision. I could see that I didn't want my dad's Tennis Club life. I could see that I might want some version of my mom's—reading famous books and writing papers about them—though I didn't want her franticness, her always having to squeeze the reading and writing in with feeding us and paying bills and having tense conversations with Dad on the front porch or on the phone.

What I could see was that writing and reading and praying and paying attention to sunrises and sunsets might somehow save me. As in, *save* me *from disappearing.*

I was deciding who I was. It was exhilarating. It was brave.

Later, I did the usual, less brave teenage stuff, like discovering how great smoking a little weed can be, now and then, for a girl whose problem is that she thinks too much. But I'm so grateful that I didn't do that at twelve or thirteen, that instead I wrote my poems and went to youth group and even stuck it out in the Girl Scouts so that I could hike. And I'm grateful that my parents either saw what was going on and chose not to try to curb my cornball tendencies—or, more likely, were so busy getting their own new lives going that they didn't notice.

Their new lives: this, really, was the unbearable thought. That my parents, whose love story had created our family, our lives—had moved on.

We already knew much more about divorce than most families, because Mom was divorced when Dad met her in 1956. Johnny and

Kristie had a different last name and a different dad, a sort of extra dad it seemed to me as a little girl, who showed up now and then on Sundays. He, that extra guy, hardly mattered when you opened the album and looked at the pictures of Mom and Dad when they were newly married: so movie-star beautiful, so clearly meant to be together!

Mom's version of the story of how she and Dad met was sort of like one of my poems in its cloud-scooping aversion to the realities of her life at the time. She had dropped out of college after a year and worked to help put her first husband through dental school. Johnny was three and Kristie was one when John left her for a woman Mom had believed was her closest friend—a fellow wife of a dental student, young and smart and fun like her. More fun, probably, since she didn't yet have children. Mom found a tiny apartment, asked her widowed Aunt Helen to come from Montana and help with the kids, and went back to work, this time as a rate clerk for Northwestern Mutual Life Insurance at Third and Pine in the heart of downtown Seattle.

One of her jobs was to train the new salesmen, most of them boys fresh out of college, just a year or two younger than she was. One of the new boys was Dad.

"He was one tall cool drink of water. Six foot three! And such a smooth talker. I just couldn't get him to leave me alone," she would say.

I used to love trying to picture this: my lanky, blond Dad in a starchy shirt and skinny fifties tie, leaning over the desk of my beautiful Mom, her dark hair swept back in a French roll like Audrey Hepburn, her sweater smooth and lipstick perfect as she punched her adding machine and rolled sheets of carbon through her typewriter and told Mike Hedreen to get back to work.

But I could never quite get Dad to reminisce like that, even when we were sitting in that very same building at Third and Pine. A few years ago, my uncle's real estate development company moved into the old Northwestern Mutual space and transformed it into a swanky, minimalist suite with concrete walls. Dad, who is semi-retired but still has a few insurance clients, keeps an office there. I viewed the move to Third and

Pine as a sign that it was time to do something I had wanted to do for years: ask Dad to talk to me on tape.

He agreed. We set a date.

The morning I arrived, nearly everyone in the office was out at a meeting. We found an empty conference room that looked more like a men's club lounge—black leather furniture, sports magazines, a big screen TV—and settled in. I turned on the tape recorder and asked Dad to tell me the story of him and Mom.

My dad is not one of those terse, reticent dads. He has a big, mellifluous voice and he loves to talk. So this was not torture for him, even though the situation—talking to his grown-up daughter about his ex-wife, now dead of Alzheimer's disease—was a little challenging. But he began.

He remembered that one day he was waiting for the bus to go to work and "quite by chance," Mom saw him and gave him a ride. And then one night they went on a double date—he and another girl and a friend of his and Mom—and they "changed partners" by the end of the evening.

"And our romance progressed and progressed and then we decided to get married," he said, by way of wrapping up.

Maybe it's just too hard, too much to ask, to go back and conjure up the magic of a marriage that ended badly forty years ago.

I asked him what Mom was like at twenty-five, when he met her. He talked about her "natural intellectual inclinations," and how much he learned from her about classical music and how even today certain pieces remind him of Mom, but then we got bogged down trying to remember the composer of the "Preludes" he was thinking of, someone Slavic but "not Dvorak": Rachmaninoff? Chopin? He talked about how she was "very domestic" and "assumed the burden of running the house," though he knew that not having finished her education was something that always frustrated her.

This was all—fine. But I wanted to hear how beautiful she was. How smitten he was. How in love they were. I wanted him to say those things without me prompting him, but he didn't.

I brought up as delicately as I could the fact that their wedding day was a little under seven months before I was born.

"We certainly were very involved with one another so you certainly could say that it could have happened but it could have gone the other way too. So I can't say. I think you want me to say, well it would have happened. But I just don't know," he said.

I can hear that now and appreciate the honesty of what he said. If I'd heard it at twelve or even twenty-five, I might have been horrified. But at fifty-three, I can look back and see all kinds of forks in the road of my own life that I could have taken, almost took, barely missed—so I do understand what Dad was trying, really honestly, to say. What if, for example, he had been accepted into the Naval Officer's Candidate program that rejected him probably, oh, not long at all before I was conceived? Would I exist? Or would I have been born on a naval base? Who knows?

Later in the interview, we talked about Mom's parents.

"The Grundstroms were somewhat of a culture shock to me," Dad said, carefully.

After Mom and Aunt Jo Ann finished high school, Grandma and Grandpa had moved from Butte, Montana to Buckley, Washington, a small farming town southeast of Seattle. It was Grandma's dream fulfilled: to get Grandpa out of the unhealthy mines, to be near her sisters, to live somewhere green. They both worked the swing shift at the state school for the mentally disabled; it was hard work but stable. They bought a few acres in the shadow of Mt. Rainier, which you couldn't see from where they were because of a thicket of trees along the fence line. Their house was a converted chicken coop and it never felt tall enough for Dad, whose loud voice and six-packs of cold beer made him popular with Grandpa and unpopular with Grandma.

I asked Dad about his first trip back to Butte when he and Mom were newly married, a road trip he took with Mom and his new in-laws. I thought he might wax on about the Rocky Mountains or have some funny memories of meeting old Finnish relatives.

But what he remembered was how few rules there were. Washingon at the time had all kinds of puritanical liquor licensing laws. Montana did not.

Dad recalled being in a bar with Mom and Grandma and Grandpa when "some nice music" came on the jukebox.

"Arlene and I enjoyed dancing," he said. So he asked the bartender if dancing was allowed. "He treated my question like it was absurd. So we danced and I was in hog heaven, having a good time and loving it."

Arlene and I enjoyed dancing.

"Some nice music" came on the jukebox.

I was in hog heaven.

It's not much, but it's something.

I can paint it. There's a shaft of light slanting in, Edward Hopper style, onto a battered wood floor and a high-backed mahogany bar with bottles on mirrored shelves and a shiny copper counter. There are just a few tables. My grandparents are at one: Grandma in a slippery flower print dress with buttons down the front, a little velveteen hat on her head; Grandpa in his brown suit and tie, his fedora on the table.

And Mom and Dad, dancing in the shaft of light. She's wearing a full, black skirt with a print that looks like cocktail olives, the one we called her gypsy skirt, and that black bateau top that showed off her sexy collarbone. Dad's in khakis and a button down shirt and a tie, because they've just been to dinner. They're dancing to Perry Como or Frank Sinatra or maybe Elvis. They're glowing with love and youth and the kind of big-city glamour that was long gone from Butte by the late 1950s, when the copper veins were all tapped out and the grim business of open pit mining had just begun to gouge the town. Everything about them says, We are the future. This old burg, that old couple sitting there, looking all worn out by the Depression? They're the past. We're young and we've got it all ahead of us: peacetime, prosperity, plenty of everything we want. And for now? Love's enough.

Our romance progressed and progressed and then we got married and it was all going to work out.

But it didn't. And I tried to ask Dad about that too.

"That's a very hard thing to discuss, particularly with you," he said. "I would say that there was—now these sound like clichés—but kind of a growing apart, an indifference to some extent, a lack of interest

54

a little bit, and then of course in my case in particular, there was this horrendous impact of meeting Maryjane, which I freely concede was a direct factor. However, it's always been my theory that if that hadn't occurred, I'm sure that things were not proceeding well. There were no dramatic fights or incidents or things of that nature but another one of my theories is that I met attractive people every day and still do today, but a good marriage has to have enough strength and attraction and so forth to withstand these things. That you can't live in kind of a sterile cocoon as it were."

Growing apart? No dramatic fights? Sterile cocoon?

The bedroom I shared with Lisa was right above my parents'. Many, many nights we lay in bed and listened to them fight. Physically fight. First we would hear talking, then yelling, then screaming, then something physical happening, then Mom sobbing and Dad slamming the door on the way out. The next day we would see bruises on her arms or legs, never her face. If she was going to play tennis and had to wear a tennis dress, she would put makeup over the bruises. Maybe those fights came after the "horrendous impact of meeting Maryjane."

The best I could muster, sitting on the black leather couch in Uncle Dick's conference room, was, "But Dad. Our room was right above yours. Your fights scared the pants off me."

He called it "arguing" and said it was "not the result of Maryjane, it was a symptom of a poor marriage." And then he talked about how they argued, for example, when they played bridge, because "You could make quite an argument: 'What do you mean, one diamond? That's a stupid bid!' So yes, there were stormy times like that and I well remember them but probably one of my psychological tricks is to try and shove them [away]—but yes, we did and I can see. One of my theories is I think it's a bad environment for children. I mean there's the one idea of holding the marriage together. But I read a great deal that this can create a lot of uncertainty in small children . . . "

And then he trailed off into a kind of magazine-style rumination full of hypothetical divorce scenarios and custody arrangements, giving me time to work up some kind of response.

"Well," I said, "I think my misfortune was to be just old enough to listen and understand, but not old enough to really know how to process it or talk about it or any of that stuff. I sometimes look back and think that's one of the reasons I got involved in religion. But also it made me very judgmental. I've laughed about it with Maryjane but as a teenager, I looked at the situation and thought, Dad's bad and adulterous and Mom's good and the victim and that's how I saw it."

"Yes," he said.

I went on. "I look back and it's too bad and I sometimes wish that you and I had been able to talk about it then. I couldn't bring it up. I was too young and shy."

"Well, I would have felt very awkward trying to verbalize it too," Dad said.

"I know," I said.

And well, that's where we left that subject.

I didn't press him about the fights and the bruises. Or about why he never explained anything to us. I didn't acknowledge that yes, Mom could be competitive.

The problem here is that I have never stopped loving my Dad. And I don't want him to stop loving me. For both of us, this interview was a huge dip into the dangerous honesty pool and I just don't know if we can swim down to the deep, deep end and I'm just not sure why we would or should, now that I'm fifty-three and he's seventy-six.

If he's reading this chapter, I hope he makes it this far. I hope he understands that the reason I will always view my parents' divorce as the first great cataclysm of my life is because I loved him then and I love him now. The hate that poured through me when I was twelve was for a grown-up world I didn't understand, a Tennis Club–world where a man could get matched with a mixed doubles partner and fall in love with her while his wife was a stone's throw away, just downhill from the tennis courts on the lovely beach, eating soft ice cream cones with his four children and two stepchildren. The hate I felt was for a world where children were expected to accept and never question what was going on between the grown-ups. A world where the father who spent one whole summer teaching me to swim could start slipping away, gradually at first—we finally taught ourselves to ride our bikes when we realized he was never going to—and then so fast that he was just gone from my daily life forever.

Or rather his whole world was gone from my daily life. And I would, forever after, only be a visitor there.

But now I had worlds of my own. I had my books and poems and guitar-strumming youth groups. I had clouds and sunsets and mountains. Divorce wasn't all bad: It had given me a chance to find these other worlds. It had given Mom a chance to finally go to college and become a teacher, to be something other than "very domestic." And Dad? He got his second try at love and marriage. He and Maryjane have been married for forty years.

The summer I was fourteen, I hiked with a group of Girl Scouts across the Olympic National Park. We carried our packs fifty miles, through the groves of thousand-year-old trees waving their crazy scarves of neon-green moss, up the hard, sweaty switchbacks, across the windy passes, into the alpine meadows full of flowers and teardrop lakes. I had never seen anything like any of it. I reveled in the old place names: Enchanted Valley, Honeymoon Meadows, Home Sweet Home, Elwha, Quinault, Duckabush, Skokomish. I lay down and stuck my head in the mountain streams and drank all the cold, clear water I wanted, something we humans can't do anymore without a filter or an iodine pill. But mostly, what stayed with me from that trip was feeling what it felt to be truly, physically strong. I walked fifty miles, carrying all my own gear. I could see the muscles in my teenaged legs. I watched my blisters turn to calluses.

We sang a lot of songs while we were backpacking, including one I still find myself humming sometimes:

I want to be strong, to be strong as the land around me
I want a heart that is wide as the sky.
I want a spirit like a moving mountain stream
I want to look people straight in the eye.

I knew who I was that summer. I knew I would never be the kind of woman who would make drinks jingle and bracelets jangle. Who could compete in a Tennis Club world. And there were times when that did feel tragic. But I knew I was strong and full of heart and spirit: I knew I could look people straight in the eye.

I hiked part of that trail recently with my husband and daughter. The old Girl Scout memories stirred and sifted, but mostly I had to focus on being strong, on carrying that load, on taking the next step. Your backpacking muscles don't quite spring to life at fifty-two the way they do at fourteen.

But doing it with Rus and Claire—it felt so much less like something that I achieved *by myself*, the way it did when I was a teen. This time, what mattered was that I was doing it with them.

And you could say that Mom was there, too. Because she helped Rus and me learn how to be parents. Because Claire looks and is so much like her and was so loved by her.

And Dad? Was he there too?

Twenty-three years ago, I came to one of those terrible forks in the road: I knew I had to leave my first husband but I had no money and no plan. Dad invited me to stay at his house. I stayed for two months. We didn't talk a lot about the details of what was going on, but he drove me to work every day, just as, forty years ago, he had driven me to junior high school every day, even though he no longer lived at our house and it was about ten miles out of his way.

Dad knew what it meant to have a second chance at love and marriage, and he helped me get mine.

Two decades later, Rus and I have sweated up a lot of switchbacks and crossed some rocky passes, but here we are, hiking the Olympics with our daughter. In a few weeks, our son will get time off from his summer job and all four of us will backpack in the North Cascades.

I can't give them the Tennis Club. But I can give them my real self.

A Hundred Christmases

There was the one who wore white patent leather loafers—in winter. There was the one who turned the faucet on when he went to the bathroom so we wouldn't hear him peeing.

There was the one who drove a Citroën and smoked pot once with Kristie.

I hated it when they left things in our house that shouldn't have been there: Cigarette butts. Whiffs of aftershave. Bottles of rye or cognac or other liquors I had never known my mother to drink.

If it had been up to me, my mom would never have engaged in anything so debasing as dating. If it had been up to me, she would have sworn off men forever, or at least for a very long time, after she and Dad divorced.

When Kristie went to college and, at fourteen, I became the oldest kid in the house, I started drinking coffee so that I could keep Mom company when she drank a cup after dinner. We brewed it Finnish-style—very strong—and drank it black.

It was the only time of day when I had her to myself. But the point was not to talk about anything deep. The point was that this was the one moment when she allowed herself to simply sit. To not hurry: to school, from school, to the store, to the stove, to the table, to her desk to grade papers or pay bills. That she seemed to enjoy my sitting with her made me feel like there was a chance I really might be growing up.

We pushed our creaky rattan-bottomed chairs back from the table and crossed our legs and blew into our big mugs. I tried to resist the temptation to tilt the chair back or clack my retainer around my mouth or twirl a strand of hair.

She told me stories about her day in the classroom: refugees from Vietnam were streaming into the junior high school where she taught, including Hmong children who had never read or written in any language, or even held a pencil. When they did begin to speak and write in English, they had tales to tell of swimming the Mekong River, walking for days, waiting in camps for relatives who never made it. Mom had done her teacher training in our neighborhood's mostly-white high school. She felt like she was swimming upstream along with her new students, trying to intuit the best ways to teach them.

She gossiped a little about the other teachers, the cranky old fossils who didn't like all these new faces or the young hipsters who tried too hard to be cool, with their caftans and guitars and peace posters: *WAR is not good for children and other living things.*

She asked me about my classes: How was sophomore English with her old friend Mr. Bass? Was he making *Romeo and Juliet* come to life? Wasn't Mercutio so much more fun than sappy old Romeo? Why on earth did Shakespeare kill him off so early in the play?

But as we sipped our coffee, the one thing we did not talk about was our own romantic lives. I still despaired of ever having one. And Mom knew better than to bring up Mr. White Shoes, or Mr. Citroën, or Mr. Faucet.

And so I don't recall exactly when Ron slipped into the mix.

I wish I'd been paying more attention. I wish I could write, *The first time Ron came by to pick Mom up for a date I immediately noticed his a) shoes b) hair c) car.* But that was the beauty of Ron: he was never one to set off alarm bells. No patent loafers, no rye whiskey.

Quite the opposite: He was a doctor, a widower with three children who belonged to the Tennis Club, though he didn't play tennis. He smoked Newport menthols and had a quiet, dry sense of humor, especially about his lack of interest in athletics. He was slim, dark-haired, thinning on top but not so much that he wasn't still classifiable as handsome. He dressed with just the right ever-so-subtle bit of flair: a blazer when other men might wear a windbreaker, Levis jeans on the weekends instead of khakis. His name was the name of a river in the

Amazon—Tocantins. TOE-kun-teens. It was one of the few names I'd come across that people mangled far more severely and frequently than Hedreen. All I knew about his family was that they came originally from Portugal, spent a generation or two in Brazil and then immigrated to the United States.

Ron married a girl from an old Philadelphia family and took her to Seattle, where he was offered a practice at a major hospital. Their children were sixteen, fourteen, and ten when his wife died of cancer.

He and Mom met at the Tennis Club bar, but he was soon taking her out to plays and the ballet and fancy benefits, the kind of social events she had never previously been anywhere near. The two of them were not head-over-heels, not at first. Ron even occasionally dated someone else, a woman he worked with whom we daughters privately referred to as The Nurse.

And then I went off to college and missed what were the best three years of their romance, when they settled into a tranquil sort of courtship that occasionally included their younger children. Lisa remembers Ron stopping by our house after he went to the supermarket on Saturday, always in his Levis and fisherman-knit sweater. James recalls playing endless games of after-dinner ping-pong with Ron's youngest son, Charles. Caroline remembers how Mom loved to stroll with Ron through his elegant old neighborhood down to the beachfront business district of Madison Park.

I do not recall my dad ever strolling with Mom.

Kristie, who was home more often than I was because she went to the University of Washington, says that with Mom and Ron, there was none of the competitive sparring that was constant in her relationship with Dad. Maybe it was because they were not raising children or running a household together.

Mom and Ron seemed able to see and hear each other in a way that Mom and Dad had forgotten, or perhaps had never learned, how to do.

Our household was very different than the Tocantins' in those years, especially at meals. At our table, everyone wanted to talk during dinner. It was hard to wait your turn. At Ron's, with his daughter Meg off at college, it was an all-male dining club: Ron; his teenaged sons Charles and Bill; and Futuro, a Japanese student who was Ron's live-in house-keeper. Whole meals went by without a word spoken.

Charles remembers how Mom liked to tell the story of her first dinner with them: "I had just lifted my second bite to my mouth," she would say, "and I looked around and saw that everyone else was finished!"

It's a funny memory, but painful. Ron shared so little with his children that Charles can't recall ever having a conversation with his dad about our mom. And yet Ron would want to stop by our house after grocery shopping, and sometimes, Charles remembered, he would sit so long chatting with Mom that the ice cream he'd just bought would melt by the time he got home.

It was an excellent time for Mom to have an easy-going relationship. In 1975, when she was in her fifth year of teaching, the strain of Seattle's early-seventies Boeing bust—more than sixty thousand people laid off, with ripple effects through hundreds of supporting businesses—finally reached the Seattle schools: voters turned down the annual school tax levy. Every teacher with less than nine years seniority was laid off. Mom's small but stable teacher's salary was replaced by occasional substitute teaching and a promise of commissions—someday—from a motiva-tional trainer. Later, she tried selling life insurance and real estate.

If she turned on the light at night and stared at the eraser smudges and carry-overs and rejuggled columns in her oversized, old-fashioned ledger, if she wondered how long she could keep this up, her daytime face was all about the power of positive thinking, or, as that motiva-tional trainer liked to say, *visualizing success.* Her letters to me were full of lines like: *Real estate can't go any lower—it's bound to start rebounding!* Everyone *needs life insurance. Subbing is great—no papers to grade!*

I had a scholarship, so her money stress didn't directly affect my college life. But I hated that she had to go through this. It seemed so outrageously unfair at a time when I was still trying to make sense of the unfairness, as my young self saw it, of divorce. Of one person simply falling out of love with another person after twelve years.

Mom had earned a B.A. and teaching certificate in seven straight quarters at the University of Washington. She got her master's degree in gifted education while she taught full time, with five children still at home. She had been a teacher for five years. How did getting laid off make any sense? Of course I understood that she wasn't alone. That there were thousands of other families like ours reeling from the Boeing layoffs and the school levy failure. But I was eighteen, so I took it very personally.

I took it personally because in order for the universe to make sense to me, I *needed* Mom to triumph. I needed her to show all those snobby, cookie-cutter, non-divorced moms—and my dad and new stepmom—that nothing was going to stop her from thriving. I wanted her to soar in a way that said, *I can be who I am and have a meaningful life; I don't need to be validated by all of you conforming social climbers.* It was a personal and emotional yearning and it was also political. And it related so politically and personally to what I wanted from my own life: success on my own terms. Genuine love: not the sad, bitter version I'd already seen too much of.

Ron fit into my What Mom Deserves scenario. Getting laid off did not. Answering phones for a motivational speaker who kept promising her "more" did not. Borrowing from her ex-husband's parents did not.

Just as, twenty years later, Alzheimer's disease would not.

Mom's financial woes did make me all the more grateful for that scholarship and for the fact that my relationship with her was not about money.

And now I had a grant to go to England my junior year: an unbelievable gift! Many of my Wellesley classmates were amused that I had never had a passport before, that I had never been *abroad*. In fact, my entire family was passport-free: neither Mom nor Dad nor any of us children had ever been further than Canada. I would be the first one of us to cross an ocean.

It was the fall of 1976. The day I arrived at the University of East Anglia in Norwich, the taxi driver dropped me on the main campus plaza, where a motley but amiable mob of black-booted students were protesting the cancellation of a Sex Pistols concert. I was elated: I could see that this year would be as unlike Wellesley as it could possibly be.

Meanwhile, Mom soldiered on with her hodgepodge of jobs. She fretted in her letters about debts and bills, but always ended optimistically: "By next spring I'll have my financial situation on a more reliable basis and, even if I have to borrow the money, I will come to see you, so be prepared!"

And then Ron offered her a Cinderella break from it all. He was going to a medical conference in Madrid. How would she like to come with him? Couldn't Kristie stay with the younger kids?

Now she too would get a passport. Cross the ocean. Leave everyday life behind.

"The trip to Spain was like a hundred Christmases all in one, like living in the middle of a fairy tale," she wrote to me afterwards. "I can't believe that life can be the same after all that, and I don't want it to be." She went on to lovingly describe the "Gothic Quarter" of Barcelona, the many "star-struck" hours she spent in the Prado while Ron was at his conference, a day-trip to Toledo that was like "stepping into the Middle Ages."

A hundred Christmases. I had been feeling that way all fall in England: the intense joy of being in a place you've imagined and read about and when you finally get there, you immediately grasp the greatest gift of all—it's not just that you're in this place, but this place is now in you, in a hundred Christmas moments of delight and discovery, all of them yours to carry in your memory, forever, to unwrap and marvel at and exclaim over again and again. And now my mom was experiencing this too, and knowing that she was—that she understood some of what I was feeling—well, that just added another Christmas or two to my own stack.

The new year brought more good luck. Mom was offered a contract job for the rest of the school year at her old school, setting up a gifted program that might or might not get continuing funding. At last, a job that would actually make use of her master's degree, an opportunity to put into practice her belief that, as she wrote in a college paper, gifted children, "as adults, armed with a healthy self-image and with their talents more fully developed, can contribute much more to a society of

64

people with many differences." Now, her paper reads a little uncomfortably, a little like a vision of a utopia for smart people. But then, what captivated her was the notion of everyone being able to live up to their potential, perhaps because she felt her own had been stymied after she dropped out of college and started having babies.

Meanwhile, she and Ron were spending more and more time together. And I was spending a lot of time with a fellow exchange student, a sweet, funny surfer from North Carolina named Dick who loved England and English literature as much as I did.

But by May, Mom's letters had begun to take on a boxing-match rhythm:

Round Two: no funding next school year for the gifted program.

Round Three: a good sales-training job offer from the phone company!

Round Four: an odd, brief "breakup" with Ron that might have had something to do with The Nurse.

Round Five: seeing more of Ron than ever.

Round Six: "Ron is suffering from double vision that seems to be connected with a sinus condition that has been causing him almost constant headaches."

Round Seven: Ron has sinus cancer.

Round Eight: Ron and I are getting married!

I missed the wedding. July 2, 1977. They felt they had to do it before Ron started treatment. I arrived home a week later, just in time to help with the move from our house to the Tocantins' house.

The radiation treatments made Ron so sick that he spent most of his time in bed. But he and Mom assured all of us that he would feel much better once the radiation was over, even though we could hear him throwing up at all hours of the night and see him shrinking inside his jeans and sweater, which he wore even on the warmest days.

Then the phone company told Mom she didn't have the right gung-ho sales attitude. She was cut from the training program.

Maybe she was just no good at selling phones. Or maybe her lack of excitement had something to do with being terribly distracted by a new marriage to a very sick husband. Or with the distractions of nine children, between the two of them, coming and going all summer.

Meanwhile, I was working nights at an Ivar's fish 'n chips restaurant and counting the days until I could see Dick again. I had finagled an affordable way to fly back to college in Massachusetts via North Carolina.

A day after I landed in Greensboro, Mom called me at Dick's parents' house. It was September second and so thickly humid—in a way that I had never experienced—that I didn't quite understand how to breathe or move.

We were in the kitchen filling Mason jar glasses with ice water when Dick's mother answered the phone.

"Ann, it's for you," she said. "Your mom. Why don't you run up and take it in your room?"

The guest room was in a corner of the house that the air conditioner seemed not to reach. I sat down on the bed and picked up the phone. The extension phone, as we used to say. My hands were clammy. I'd left my water downstairs.

"Mom?"

"Oh, honey," Mom said. "I don't know how to tell you this but I'm exhausted so I'll just tell you."

Sweat was running in a stream between my breasts.

"Ron died last night."

Now I really couldn't breathe. My heart was starting to pump desperately as if it couldn't find oxygen.

Mom was saying more. Words like *quickly, no idea, shock.*

There were black spots dancing in the room.

"Mom, I want to come home. I want to be there."

She said she didn't want me to come home. It would cost too much and she didn't want me to miss school. She said she had to go, that she had to get through so many more calls, that we'd talk soon.

When I hung up the phone, I stood up too fast and almost fainted. There was nowhere in Dick's house to breathe! How could anyone live in this awful, unbreathable air! I was crying but it felt more like gasping.

I wanted so much to be home that very minute, to put my arms around Mom, do something for her, anything.

It still seems so strange to me that I didn't go home. Neither did Lisa, from her college in California. But it was a different era in our family history. Death was not something we knew. Grieving was not something we knew. And no one had any money for our plane tickets.

But it meant that, during the darkest time of my mother's life that I had ever known, darker even than her divorce from Dad, I wasn't there: to make her coffee after dinner or go to the grocery store or hang out with Jimmy and Caroline and Charles or whatever she wanted me to do. It meant that I had to wait three months before I could finally hug her.

It was hard to believe that I had been so worked up about the school levy failure and its shocking unfairness. Now Mom was on some cosmic slide, some divine lab test in which she was the guinea pig: just how much unfairness can one person take? Ron's three children seemed to be part of the same experiment: first their mother, now their father?

"She was never the same," we love to intone dramatically when describing a survivor of tragedy. One would hope so. What would be shocking is if someone *was* the same. Mom was swimming her own Mekong River now: getting laid off; getting married; getting laid off again; losing her new husband; gaining three orphaned stepchildren, one of them still in high school—all in a handful of months.

May. June. July. August. September.

"If love be rough with you, be rough with love," said clever, doomed Mercutio. Love had been rough with Mom all right. Love delivered the knockout blow and walked away from the ring. Left her bleeding and bruised and alone.

Left her *in the middle of it all*, as the R&B song goes:

But I wonder what my friends would say.
If their world just came down one day.
And they were in the middle of it all.

Caroline, who was twelve at the time, knew Mom sometimes stayed in bed all day while she and James and Charles were at school. James, who was fourteen, said she kept up a good front: she made conversation, she cooked dinner every night. But he remembers once being in the car with her when "Fire and Rain" came on the radio and she began to cry and he didn't know what to say.

Charles was a senior in high school. Suddenly his father was dead, his brother and sister were back on the East Coast, Futuro had gone back to Japan, and his new housemates were Arlene and her two adolescent children.

"The only thing I knew how to do was what my dad had always done," Charles said. "Not talk about it."

He remembers going to dinner that fall at a family friend's, wandering upstairs and opening a door, only to find Mom sobbing her heart out in the arms of their hostess. He closed the door quickly. Never talked about it.

He remembers Mom saying, some years later, that even though Ron never told her he loved her, she knew that he did.

For Charles and James and Caroline, the fall of 1977 was a surreal and disorienting season. But at least they had school. They had their daily routine. Charles drove his new stepbrother and stepsister to their junior high every morning.

For Mom, that fall must have felt so terrifyingly empty. She wasn't working, though she knew she would have to start soon: Ron had left her in charge of a large house and a rapidly shrinking bank account. She was alone in the house all day, a house full of another family's things. She took to wearing Ron's fisherman sweater.

A year and a half after Ron's death, Mom wrote an impassioned letter to the Seattle School District about how much she loved teaching and deserved to be rehired. "I have continued as a substitute teacher for many reasons, the craziest of which is that I really want to teach in Seattle, where my six children have all attended school, because I think the district needs teachers with my energy, qualities, and dedication," she wrote.

The district moved her up from daily sub to a succession of long-term fill-in gigs: maternity leaves, medical leaves, sabbaticals.

At last, in 1985, she landed and stayed for five straight years at the school she loved best of all: her children's alma mater, Roosevelt High School.

It was a good stretch. Until her brain began to betray her. With little scratches, at first, "not so deep as a well, nor so wide as a church door."

But, like Mercutio's mortal wound, they were enough; they served.

"I used to think I could do anything I wanted to do," Mom wrote on a page torn from a notebook she kept for a few weeks in the summer of 1984. "I think I still believe that, in spite of all the evidence to the contrary. But what do I want? I think I truly desire to experience serenity and contentment in solitude . . . maybe I'm not meant to be alone. However, alone I will be frequently, and I must learn to do more than just deal with it. I want to enjoy creatively that time alone."

She made a list of goals: financial, social, weight, exercise, art, "writing for personal satisfaction and profit." She thought she might write "anecdotal advice to single parents and older women suddenly found alone." That was item number three on her writing-idea list. Number two was short stories. Number one was her mother's story: "from her parents' emigration to living at Parkside," the retirement home where Grandma Cere spent her final year. It would be, Mom wrote, "an exploration of her experiences/character/milieus/friends/associates/family from her daughter's very subjective viewpoint."

It's just a scribbled page ripped from a wirebound notebook: a page that looked like it had been crumpled and thrown away, and then uncrumpled and tucked in the same file where she kept her will.

As if she wanted us to know what she would have done. What she had meant to do.

Sisu

Dr. Forsythe was a neurologist who had tested Mom; he was not her regular doctor. His office, lined with bookshelves, felt more like a professor's than a physician's. He looked like a professor too, with his goatee and crossed legs and large, expressive hands. I'm not sure what my siblings and I were hoping for when we requested a meeting with him. Hope, I suppose, some special brand of hope that could not be transmitted over the phone but could only be dispensed in person. By him. To us.

And so there we were, Kristie, Mom, and me, sitting across an unnaturally tidy desk from the bearded doctor, our knees pressed together, our faces upturned, like three polite co-eds asking for an extension on a term-paper deadline.

Dr. Forsythe began by saying a lot of encouraging things about Mom's brightness and competence and how her intellectual skills would help her cope.

He talked about having confirmed, through three screenings over five years, her brain's "slow deterioration." He talked about medications that might slow some of the symptoms of a "dementia such as Alzheimer's disease." He talked about considering moving from her home to somewhere safer.

He avoided saying the exact words, "You have Alzheimer's disease." But he came as close as he could.

It was a warm day, for June. My mind wandered to the wool sweater vest Dr. Forsythe was wearing under his white lab coat. The vest looked itchy and lumpy and homemade. Maybe his mother knit it for him and he was going to meet her for lunch.

I put my pen away because I could see that Kristie was taking plenty of notes. I noticed how pretty Mom looked, her face animated as she listened to Dr. Forsythe.

But mostly I felt like I could not wait to get away from this stuffy office, from the doctor's kind voice, from Kristie and her notes, from Mom and her stoic calm.

I wanted to get away because I was having the one thought I knew I should not be having at such a moment: *I'm not up to this. Whatever this is.*

Claire's eighth birthday was a few days away. I was about to host a slumber party for a dozen eight-year-old girls. *That* I was up to. I was concerned about Rus—he'd been working too hard; he seemed brittle and distracted. That, too, I was surely up to. But this talk of deterioration and dementia and safety and moving; these notes that Kristie was furiously scribbling; this notion that our mom, of all people, was headed down some sort of grim path that ended in—in what? Drooling in a wheelchair?

No. This I was not up to.

Perhaps my face was projecting this heresy. Dr. Forsythe offered to summarize the meeting in a letter to Mom, with copies to Kristie and me.

In his single-spaced, nearly two-page letter, he gently explained his findings, such as, "By far the major difficulty is in new learning and memory functions . . . It appears that it is extremely difficult to maintain newly experienced information over a time period of say fifteen to twenty minutes or so," and "We have no way of knowing really the course of future deterioration, but I suspect that the best estimate is that things may continue to very slowly change over the years." Dr. Forsythe concluded by saying, "I am quite impressed with your strength, honesty, and determination in dealing with the stresses this illness has brought upon you. I am also quite impressed by your very supportive family."

Things may continue to very slowly change . . . your strength, honesty, and determination . . . your very supportive family.

I wish I could ask Mom's forgiveness for not being very supportive that afternoon.

For not even rallying the way I did the first time she rode the chairlift to the top of the ski area and I, her partner, at all of about eleven years old, found myself saying things like, "Mom! Think of sitting at a chair at the dinner table. The one thing you never do is fall off your chair, right?"

There she was, all strength, honesty, and determination, not anywhere near falling off her chair while a neurologist in a sweater vest talked about her "future deterioration" and I, her grownup daughter, couldn't wait to go buy slumber-party snacks.

Why is it that we talk about illness as if we're at war? The obituary pages are full of people who waged long battles, courageous struggles, fought hard, never gave up. But it's not like anyone ever wins, so why do we pretend that they might have? If only—what? If only they'd fought harder?

Strength. Honesty. Determination.

When Mom was diagnosed with probable Alzheimer's disease, most people had no idea what to say. But some people started talking to her like she'd just been drafted. "Tough luck, the worst, but you're so smart, Arlene, you can fight this thing." To us, they'd say things like, "Your mom is one tough cookie. She's not going to take this lying down."

Lots of people wanted to help her choose her weapons: crossword puzzles, blueberries, Gingko, Vitamin E, green tea, red wine, exercise.

Others recommended defensive fortifications: hide-a-keys, ID bracelets, timers on outdoor lights, daughters on speed dial.

Loyal friends took on a USO role, keeping regular, morale-boosting dates for dinners and plays and concerts. We, her children and grandchildren, were sometimes R&R and sometimes the backup support troops: the drivers, bursars, provisioners, strategists, medical officers.

But many, many hours of every day and night, she was by herself, walking a dark and lonely vigil. She knew this wasn't some "battle" she could "win." And I wonder what those private moments, when she didn't have to pretend to be tough, when there were no witnesses—I wonder what those moments were like.

I don't know.

I'm sure there were many that she never told us about. Either because she really didn't remember, or because she did and she knew how pathetic it would sound to us.

One day I stopped by her house and saw that her arm was black and blue.

"Oh, it was just a little slip down the stairs," she said. "You know how easily I bruise."

It didn't look like a little slip. It looked more like she'd tumbled all the way down the stairs and landed hard on her arm, maybe because she had forgotten the stairs were there.

And yet that moment of landing at the bottom of the stairs, *in that moment* surely she felt terrified: What had just happened? What had her brain just done, or rather not done?

When our son Nick was born in April 1992, Mom had just decided to retire from teaching a year early. I viewed the situation entirely self-ishly: now she could be my part-time daycare. I told myself it wasn't really all about me, that Mom loved babies, was great with babies, had told me she wanted to do it. I told myself there was no danger in it, that being unable to quote Shakespeare to teenagers the way she used to did not disqualify her as a loving grandma and babysitter.

But a pattern was starting to develop, a pattern of there being no pattern.

I would arrive excited to see Nick and brimming over with breast milk. One of my great pleasures, when Claire was a baby, had been this moment of arriving at her daycare and swooping her up and sitting right down to feed her. But with Mom, I could not count on this happening. She couldn't remember *not* to feed him, even though she was proud of having breast-fed six children back when it wasn't the fashion.

I tried leaving notes. I tried calling her and reminding her. But still, I would show up at three thirty, after fetching Claire from preschool, and there they would be: Mom, Nick, and an empty bottle, looking at me guiltily from the couch.

"But he was hungry," she would say. "And he's such a good eater, and you know there's just no stopping him once you start. And—I'm never quite sure when you're coming."

"Mom, I come at the same time every day," I would say. "It's not such a long time, from lunch to three thirty. But if he's really hungry you're supposed to call me, remember?"

I knew how much she loved her time with Nick; I knew he made her feel young again, like he was her little boy. I knew she wheeled him around the neighborhood and all the shopkeepers and neighbors admired him—but why couldn't she remember what it was like to be full of milk, dying to feed your baby? Knowing you'd have to go home and use the dreaded breast pump, while wrangling a baby and a three-year-old?

I remember one day walking in and seeing Nick, full and happy, and the bottle empty and feeling the pain in my breasts and bursting into tears and saying, "I'm sorry Mom, I know it's hard to remember stuff but this is really hard for me." I cried all the way home, Claire and Nick looking at me, puzzled, from their car seats. I remember knowing that I wasn't really crying about the milk and the pain and the hated pump. I was crying because I had looked forward so much to this time with Mom, this time when she would be a young grandma and I would be a young mom and we'd have such great conversations and memorable shared moments. But it wasn't like that. Something was wrong with her. Not only could she not remember not to feed Nick, she couldn't remember the plot of a book or a movie or what we were talking about five minutes ago.

I was crying, that day in the car, because I was already starting to miss her, even though that made no sense, since she was right there.

Maybe she cried too, after I left. She must have missed herself as much as I did: the Arlene who once upon a time could remember a thousand things, who read Tolstoy while she nursed her babies, who couldn't imagine how Anna Karenina could leave her child.

I wonder whether it was worse for her before or after she knew what it was that was slowly strangling her brain.

Ten years before the June day in 1997 when Dr. Forsythe gave her the deliberately not quite definitive diagnosis—because it never is, with Alzheimer's disease, not until after death—she had started to talk about those moments in front of the classroom. For ten years—a decade that included her retirement, three of her children's weddings, the births of eight of her fourteen grandkids—she had been aware that her brain was slipping in a way that she guessed, correctly, was much more serious than the little moments her friends were starting to report. Yet until that summer afternoon in 1997, she could still hope that it was something chronic, something annoying, something to be lived with, that these memory lapses were her concession to aging, like the tennis elbow or arthritis that plagued some of her peers.

I can picture her after the appointment, after Kristie and I have dropped her off. She's alone again, walking into her quiet, modern house with its walls of east-facing windows, hanging her jacket and silk scarf in the hall closet and going into the kitchen for . . . tea? Or wine?

She's disappointed that Kristie and I can't stop in, that we have kids to pick up and work to get back to. Or maybe she's glad to be alone.

She reaches for a glass and opens the fridge and uncorks the white wine and says to herself, *Oh, why not.*

She sits down at the kitchen table and takes that first cold sip and looks out at the lake where, far below, a cluster of tiny sailboats is careening around in a strong wind.

She suddenly feels—expendable.

Expendable, she says to herself. *That's a word Dr. Forsythe would like to hear me use. "See, Arlene? With a vocabulary like that, you're way ahead in this battle!"*

Was she plucky like that, when she was by herself? That's how she was with us. If we had been there, she would have joked about how it was too bad she preferred white wine, since red was supposed to be good for your brain. She would have pointed out the boats, and reached for her camera to take a picture of them.

It's hard to imagine her thinking of suicide. She wasn't the type. She prided herself on her *sisu*, the secret toughness possessed only by the Finnish people. Strength. Honesty. Determination.

But, in that moment, did the thought cross her mind?

The sailboats are bumping into each other, a beginner's class. Mt. Rainier is in the clouds one minute, dramatically visible the next. Maybe the sailors are distracted by the mountain.

How would she have done it? Pills?

No. Because she couldn't control who would discover her, and what if it was me and Claire and Nick were with me? What if it was Caroline or James or Lisa, whose children were even younger than mine?

That cold wine tastes good. She pours herself another glass. After all, who's there to see her, to watch her brain wasting away?

The smartest girl in Butte High School. She used to tell us that, proudly; now she says it to herself wistfully. Her comeuppance at last: Alzheimer's.

The phone rings.

She considers not answering it. But then she thinks, *No, I better. I hate to think the kids are going to worry even more now.*

"Hello? Caroline! Hi, sweetie. I'm fine. Oh, that. Well, it's not the greatest news, is it, but at least now we all know why I've been so batty. A group? What sort of a group? Oh honey, you know I'm not a joiner. Oh, I see, it's more of a class. Well yes, let's do that then. OK then. Yes, I'm putting it on my calendar now. OK, talk to you soon."

She hangs up the phone and reaches for a pen, but the sun is just breaking over the top of one of the clouds and she has to watch it, it's too beautiful, it's like a Tiepolo ceiling, and by the time she reaches for her date book she's forgotten when the class is.

It's OK. Caroline will call and remind her. Even though she doesn't really see why she should take a class and hear all about Alzheimer's when she's the one who has it and already knows more about it than she wants to know. But Caroline seems to really want her to do it, so she'll do it. If it will make her kids feel better, she'll do these things for them.

That's it, really, she thinks. She's got to show that sisu. For her kids and grandkids.

But in the meantime, why not just drink a little more wine and take in the mountain and the clouds and the lake for about five more minutes. *Five more minutes.*

Those crazy little sailboats. She never really did understand the appeal of trying to make a boat go where you want it to by pulling this rope or that rope and hoping you'll catch the right breeze at the right moment. Paddling a canoe, rowing a rowboat—that was more her style. Off you go, under your own steam, enjoying the view along the way instead of wrapping yourself up in a big tangle of ropes.

The Madrona House

Mom had never lived in a house that didn't come with all the baggage of a man attached to it.

But the Madrona house was different. This house was hers. She chose it. She paid for it. Only she lived in it. It was just the right size and you could see the lake and the mountains and it was on a steep hillside so no one walking on the street below could see her, sitting in bed with her cereal and her crossword. And it was in the perfect neighborhood: Madrona, a cluster of old bungalows and brick Tudors and boxy Queen Annes settled like moss on a steep Seattle hill thirty blocks due east of downtown and just above Lake Washington. Tucked here and there were a few modestly modern, sixties-era cliff-hangers built to blend in, not stand out. The house she bought was one of those.

This home would hold no memories of dying husbands, ex-husbands, her father's hacking miner's cough. This house would be hers to paint in buttery colors and to furnish with graceful pieces: a striped couch stretched out in a long, clean arabesque; a highly polished table like a bare, spotlit stage. It would be hers to fill with a whole wall of bookshelves and an easel and an exercise bike downstairs and no bookshelves, no clutter, upstairs. Hers to arrange with no regard for the needs of messy children and careless men. Her front door to open when she wished.

She was fifty-two years old when she bought the Madrona house. She had been raising children since she was just out of her teens. Ron's children were heartbroken and angry when she sold their father's baronial home—but Mom was a schoolteacher, she couldn't afford to keep it up, and they all lived far from Seattle and showed no signs of coming back any time soon. She gave them what she thought was a fair settlement. She saw her far more humble new house, with its nearly identical view of the mountains and the lake, as an homage to the life she had briefly shared with their father, though they didn't see it that way. How could they?

And now I am fifty-three. And in all my adult life—no, in all my whole life—I have lived alone for no more than a few months at a time. There was my junior year in college, when I had a single dorm room; there were the seven or so months I spent in a studio apartment after I left Dick and before Rus moved in with me.

I could pretend that I have had more control over where I've lived than Mom did: I am a working partner, wife, mother; I waited until I was thirty-two to have children. But Dick and I lived together not just because we were young and in love but because we were too poor to live apart. And Rus moved in with me after we got back from Haiti so that we could save money for a long honeymoon.

So when I think of Mom, at fifty-two, finally giving up on caretaking a house that was never hers, that was a museum of grief for her dead husband and his elegant first wife—finally giving it up for a house that was plain and sunny and *all* hers—I can well imagine the relief and freedom and joy she must have felt. And when I think of her sixteen years later being told by her uppity children that she had to, *had to* move out, I can imagine her sorrow and rage.

She knew that Alzheimer's disease was eating her memory. She had known it, on some level, since before she went to Haiti. But, she tried to reason with us, with all the reason she still had: wouldn't leaving this house she loved and had lived alone in for—well, who cares exactly how many years, she would say, but way more than ten—wouldn't that just make it harder for her? She acknowledged the falls down the stairs—the "little slips" as she called them, even though they left bruises like ugly thunderclouds—the burner left on that turned the copper tea kettle coal black, the garage door left open like a gaping mouth. But she tried to persuade us that these incidents were not dangerous but silly, just bumps in the road of her daily life, just like all of our childhood skinned knees and stepped-on nails and bee stings and broken bones. The stairs, the burner, forgetting the keys—they're just dumb stuff, she would say, the things that everyone does whether or not they have Alzheimer's. No more dangerous than crossing the street.

And, she might add, what about holidays? Where would we gather on Christmas Day, Thanksgiving, Easter, if there were no Madrona house?

We have homes now, Mom, we would say. We're not in apartments and dorms any more. And besides—but this part we said only to each other—watching Mom try to orchestrate the holiday meal was becoming more nerve-wracking than doing it ourselves. Even if we brought almost everything and did almost everything, her moment-to-moment inability to remember gave our holidays a sort of manic, surrealist theatre flavor:

"Let's see, how about the gravy?"

"Done, Mom, it's on the table."

"OK, great. Now how about the gravy?"

Our children remember the Madrona house differently. It was the house where they opened Christmas presents, hunted for Easter eggs, played with their cousins: games like Pig Pile on Matthew (the oldest cousin), or Sardines (like Hide 'n Seek except only one person hides and everyone else seeks and when you find the hider, you crawl in too), or the game of seeing who could untie the most grownups' shoes under the table before getting caught. When they were shooed out of the dining room, they went downstairs and cycled away on Grandma's exercycle, tossed around our beat-up old toys—sad stuffed animals and dingy ABC blocks—or watched one of Grandma's half dozen movies: *Annie*, *West Side Story*, *Fiddler on the Roof*, the old Mary Martin TV version of *Peter Pan*. For them, it was the center of the family universe.

And in the decade since Mom left the Madrona house, we haven't had a center. There are too many of us, and we're too conscientious about taking turns.

As we slowly coaxed her into looking at retirement complexes, my sisters and I grumbled to each other about Mom's rejection of all apartments with views inferior to the view from the Madrona house. But we knew it was much more than that. We knew it was about leaving the one place she had ever lived that was truly hers. We knew it was about having started life in a dozen different Finntown tenement flats in Butte, Montana, each one smaller than the one before, until finally, with every penny gone, no work in sight, and the Depression at its worst, Grandpa had to go to his sour, arrogant brother-in-law and beg for shelter for his wife and little girls. Mom had friends in apartments and condos but she always swore she would never live stacked up with other people again.

And now we were asking her to live stacked up with what looked and felt, to all of us, like a lot of people twenty years older than her.

"They all use those THINGS!" she said, the word "walker" eluding her.

The Finntown tenements: by the time I saw them on my first trip to Butte when I was twelve, most of them were gone and the ones that were left were half-empty. But they looked just as Mom had described them, with their criss-crossing, rickety back stairs and the long hallways tunneling through the buildings just like the mine shafts that went right under the neighborhood. Mom's cranky old landlord, Uncle Albert, was long gone, but her sweet Auntie Helen still lived there and still wore the same button-down print dresses and black lace shoes that she wore in all the old photo albums.

Mom used to tell us that she moved so many times as a child she lost count. Often, it wasn't called "moving." Her parents would say, "We're going to visit Grandma for a while." Or, "We're going to visit Auntie Helen." Or, "We're going to go camping for the whole summer and eat fried trout and cornmeal mush every day!"

Those were the kinds of memories Mom always said she wanted to write down. She started to, in some of the classes she took when she went back to college. I know about Uncle Albert, who died before I was born, because she wrote a scathing character sketch of him, sitting in the same chair all day in his one-piece union suit and overalls, spitting tobacco in a can, while Helen waited on him and his tenants brought him their rents or their excuses. She also wrote a story about going out on her first blind date at forty and debating whether to tell the man, whom she described as a "Swedish shipping magnate," that she had six children. Her professors wrote comments on her papers like, "Great start, Arlene, but I feel you rushed to the finish line," which I'm sure she did, with all of us underfoot and the rest of her homework to do.

And then, in the Madrona house, when at last she wasn't rushing anymore—it was suddenly too late to write it all down. The finish line and the starting line too had gotten lost in the big, knotted-up net of her brain.

But she could still tell her stories, and a few became trusted conversational friends that she pulled out when Alzheimer's left her high and dry.

"People think you can't remember anything," she would quip. "That's not true. I remember all kinds of things. Just never in the right order or at the right time!" And then she would go on about how she could remember making mud pies with her sister in Butte, Montana like it was yesterday, explaining that they had to play in the dirt because there was no grass in Butte: not a blade, at least not in Finntown. Nothing grew there. It may have been the richest hill on earth but to a little girl, it was dirt and soot and, three times a day, streets filled with great crowds of men, half of them covered in dirt and the other half clean.

Then she would remind us how lucky we were, having grown up surrounded by green, how growing up in Butte, green was not a color she missed because it was a color she didn't think of as part of her everyday life. It was a color she visited: at the Columbia Gardens on Sundays. Or in the summertime when she went camping with her family or with the Girl Scouts.

"But," she would continue, "We sure knew the color white back in Butte. You don't know what snow is here in Seattle!" She and her sister had loved how the snow made the Butte streets magic and beautiful, at least for a few hours, before the trolleys and cars and miners' footsteps mucked it up. Once it snowed in June and the city shut down for a day because all the plows had been put away.

"Imagine that," Mom would say, "we schoolkids had a snow day in June. We threw snowballs in June!"

She loved the story of the snow day in June. But often it made her wistful and led right into the Berkeley Pit story. "Now all anyone can see in Butte is the Pit," she would say with a sigh. "The Berkeley Pit, the biggest open-pit mine in America. Maybe you've heard of it. It's where all those migrating swans landed and died a couple years ago, because they drank the water and it was full of poison."

She could keep it going, during the Madrona house years. And I would ache because they were good stories, but I'd heard them all. And maybe I'd been alone with my tiny children all weekend, maybe Rus was out of town and I was dying to talk, to have a conversation, but listening to Mom's old stories wasn't a conversation.

Or maybe I wasn't dying to talk at all, I wanted to get home and get some work or writing or reading done but I was trapped by the mud pie story or the snow day in June story and I felt miserable and hateful and guilty because Mom had just given me some precious babysitting time and I didn't have the patience to sit still, again, for her stories.

I became obsessed, during those years when she did a lot of babysitting for me, with the distance between her house and mine: 5.2 miles. Five point two miles up the lake and up the hill, from my jumbled neighborhood of weirdly remodeled ranch houses and Cape Cods to lovely, mossy Madrona. It took about fifteen minutes to drive it. That would be thirty round-trip. But time was so scarce, with young children and freelance work, that I fantasized about how much more time I would have if only I lived in Mom's neighborhood and wasn't always driving back and forth. But we couldn't afford her neighborhood and I felt like a materialistic pig for even wishing we could, just like I felt like an impatient baby for not wanting to listen to her same old stories. And yet I also felt trapped by the whole arrangement. I didn't make enough money to justify finding and paying for daycare closer to home. Besides, how do you fire your mom? And Rus thought I was being ridiculous, complaining about the drive. He loved our house for many good reasons, including the fact that it was fifteen minutes closer to the airport than Mom's. He was freelancing for CBS and flying a lot.

So up and down the lake I drove: taking Claire to preschool, dropping Nick at Mom's, coming home for two or three or four hours, depending on what day it was, and then turning around and doing it all again.

Looking back, it's clear to me now that the problem was not the drive. The problem was that I was achingly lonely, especially when Rus was out of town. I missed him, I missed working with him, I missed having a real job with real work friends, I missed my grownup self and my grownup mind. I felt like I couldn't befriend other stay-at-home moms because I had my freelance work to do and my writing and so little time.

I felt guilty in every possible way: guilty for not making friends with the preschool moms, who probably, rightfully, thought I was arrogant and standoffish; guilty that I wished I could bond with them, that my two children weren't enough; guilty for not being more grateful to Rus for his willingness to earn most of our income; guilty for not being more grateful that I had a Mom who wanted to babysit.

But that was the other big part of my loneliness, though I don't think I quite got this until many years later: I missed Mom. I missed the Mom we'd seen in Haiti, despite that one strange evening.

I missed the Mom who, seven months later, had skipped a week of school and come all the way to Scotland to attend our humble wedding and wish us well as we set off with our backpacks and round-the-world plane tickets on an extended honeymoon that most of our other relatives didn't know what to make of (*They're leaving their good jobs? To do what?*), but Mom understood, she got it, she knew that traveling together would make us rich in a way that a year's worth of paychecks never could. I missed the Mom who threw us a big party at the Madrona house for our first anniversary and laughed harder than anyone when one of our friends, who didn't know her neighborhood, bushwhacked up the steep hill below her house, burst into the living room via the deck, his shoes covered with mud, and promptly belted out "Danny Boy" in our honor. I missed the Mom who could never quite understand why I didn't love a good crossword like she did but was always happy to play me at Scrabble and, more often than not, beat me.

I missed the Mom I thought I was going to get so much of during this time in our lives, hanging out with her at her Madrona house.

Instead I was getting mud pies, nothing green, snow days in June, the swans who died in the Berkeley Pit and 5.2 miles, over and over again.

And when things started to get scarier—with the falls down the stairs and the lockouts and the burners left on and the word: *Alzheimer's*—then I felt so guilty for missing her. For wanting her to be what she could no longer be.

One Saturday in April 1999, not long after her sixty-eighth birthday, we moved Mom from the Madrona house to an assisted living apartment at the Lakeview retirement community. It was a balletic day: my brothers-in-law Pat and Marty jeté-ing up and down the lake in their pickup trucks; the rest of us loading them up in Madrona, unloading them at the Lakeview, trying not to bump into each other; Mom enjoying her directorial role as we arranged and re-arranged her new home.

I know she felt lucky to have so many children to help with the move. But how did it feel after we'd all gone, to sit there that first evening on her beloved striped couch, now squeezed into a shoebox of a living room?

She didn't have a view of the lake after all: she had a view of the front parking lot. A lakeside apartment would open up soon, we were assured, and Mom would get it. But meanwhile, she had a view of cars, though none of them were hers, because she'd turned in her license. And she had a view of the front door, where people her age came and went, visiting their ninety-year-old parents.

Maybe it felt a little like our house after Dad left: calmer, but dull and lonely. After he moved out, she had told me that sure, it was nice to have some peace, but she still felt like someone had cut off her arm. I was the kind of preteen girl who wouldn't watch bloody movies and the vividness of that image stayed with me forever.

This time, it was she who had been amputated: From her life as she had known it. From the home that had been hers for sixteen years, the longest she ever lived anywhere.

I walked past the Madrona house a few days ago. I don't think Mom would like the new olive green paint job with the black trim. But the cherry tree she planted on the steep slope below has grown up. It was putting on quite a blossomy show. Across the street, an old rhododendron was blooming early, its flowers the very palest, pearliest shade of pink, as if it wanted to be a cherry tree too, even if it meant having nothing left at all by May.

The air was unusually dry, warm for March, more Rocky Mountains than wet Seattle. You could almost imagine the smell of Ponderosa pines. The clarity of that dry, piney scent.

On that first Montana trip when I was twelve, Mom took me and ten-year-old Lisa horseback riding one afternoon at an old stable outside of Butte. It was the same stable where Mom and her friends used to ride after school: twenty-five cents an hour for a mountain-air break from the smokestacks and sooty streets of Butte.

Lisa and I had been on a horse maybe twice in our lives. We were still fumbling and panicking and trying to get our reins and stirrups organized when Mom suddenly turned her horse and took off up the trail at a brisk trot.

"Back in a few minutes," she called over her shoulder. "You'll be fine!"

We were stunned: first, that our mother actually knew how to do this; second, that she was leaving us behind.

By the time she came back, we still had not made it out of the corral. But we could see that she had been—somewhere. That she had taken a break from us. Gone somewhere that her mind needed and wanted to go in that newly single summer of her life.

Her face looked different, like she knew what longing was, what aching was—the same kind of longing and aching that I was just beginning to know, at twelve. I understood, for the first time, that her own mind might sometimes be as full to bursting as my own, full of her own daydreams and desires and hopes for the future—but on that afternoon, lucky her, she had been able to relieve the pressure with a ride up the trail under a pine-dry Montana sky.

At the Lakeview, she was trapped. Madrona had been such a great neighborhood for walking. Now, the only trail she could see from her window was a crosswalk that led from her side of Rainier Avenue to a cluster of businesses on the other. One was a convenience store that bore the name, "Why? Grocery."

In those early months in her new home, Mom made many trips to the "Why?" There was nowhere else to go. You'd think there might have been a pleasant path down to the lake, but there wasn't: the Lakeview had a lake view, but no lake shore.

Mom began to talk about Montana even more often. She yearned to make one more trip. But it would have been up to one of us to make that happen, and somehow the time just galloped away.

I look back and I marvel at how I slackened the reins and just wantonly, recklessly *allowed* the time to gallop. Never slowing down enough to ask the right questions:

Why no lake path at the Lakeview?

Why couldn't I carve out a week, one tiny week of my life, and take Mom to see Butte again?

And why the "Why? Grocery"?

The Troubles

There's a snapshot I keep in my mind, a moment of being surprised by one of those sudden downpours of pure joy: I am walking, almost running with eagerness, towards the Boiserie Café on the University of Washington campus on an urgently bright summer day and I see my mom, holding my three-month-old son, smiling and waving at me. Both of them are smiling; Nick is still too young to properly wave but as soon as he sees me he does the baby version, wildly wiggling his arms and legs and bottom. Mom, too, in my snapshot-memory, seems to be smiling and waving with her whole self, spilling her smile, her love, all over the outdoor tables full of languorous summer students. And then Mom and I are laughing at Nick's crazy wiggle as she hands him to me and we sit down at a table under a chestnut tree where I can nurse and we can drink iced mochas and eat a couple of the Boiserie's amazing raspberry mazurka bars. I was bottomlessly hungry that summer.

It was July of 1992 and Mom had just retired from teaching. She was taking an oil painting class on campus; I was taking African Art History because there was a chance that Rus and I might be doing a documentary on the Seattle Art Museum's unusual African collection. Two days a week, our classes lined up so that Mom could watch Nick during mine and then I could take over in time for her to head to the painting studio.

We were both drunk with love for the same things that summer: for baby Nick, mainly, but also for art and for the sudden bestowing of time—her retirement, my maternity leave—and for summer itself, Seattle's benign, breezy, green season of days that are more like perfect spring days in any other city.

Eighteen years later, that portrait of smiling Mom and smiling Nick now seems the embodiment of all innocence: both of them so full of everyday, small-"j" joy; neither of them knowing that Nick would be the last baby to be trusted, without hesitation, to her care and love.

Of course, you're thinking. *Alzheimer's disease.* Yes. It breaks my heart to see Mom in my mind, then, and to know what the next five years, ten years, fourteen years in all would be like for her.

But there was another heartbreak waiting, and this one was mine.

In the gallows-humor retelling of this story, I sometimes start right off by laying the blame on Tonya Harding. Maybe you've forgotten Tonya: she was the bad-girl ice skater from the wrong side of the tracks—charm-challenged Clackamas County, Oregon, just upriver from charming Portland—whose boyfriend kneecapped her good-girl rival, Nancy Kerrigan. Tonya entered my life, our lives, when Rus got a call from CBS to go to Portland and cover her court hearing.

"You'll be home tonight," the L.A. bureau chief said.

Thirty-five days later, thirty-five straight days in union talk, Rus had made more than $30,000 and Nick, Claire, and I had made two weekend visits to Portland on the CBS dime because the bureau chief couldn't let Rus leave in case Tonya did one more nutty thing. Connie Chung had flown out to Portland and kissed Rus and his sound man Pat after her interview with Tonya for *48 Hours.* I had bought a stack of short story collections from Powell's bookstore because I was now taking an evening series of creative writing classes. The story I was working on was about a young mom who runs away from home. And Rus, during his many days of standing around in courtroom hallways, had come up with an idea of what to do with the Tonya Harding windfall.

"I'm going to make a movie," he said to me over Thai crab cakes in our Portland hotel suite. "A short feature. I have a script I've been working on. And I can use the Tonya money to hire a real crew and shoot in sixteen-millimeter."

My own bourgeois mind had already imagined that $30,000 as a down payment on a house in my mom's neighborhood. Or if not that, then maybe we could remodel our concrete tomb of a basement. But I was in a new marital position: financially powerless. I made a few thousand dollars a year doing freelance PR, mostly for art museums. Rus had just made $30,000 in a little over a month. And even though it was supposed to be our money—his travel for CBS made possible by my willingness to stay home—we both knew it wasn't.

Besides, his CBS work made it possible for me to take writing classes and pursue my creative dream. What right did I have to object to Rus pursuing his? For a decade, he had been shooting news and dreaming of making a real movie.

And so Tonya Harding financed his film, as he later wrote in a column for a movie magazine. And in so doing, Tonya launched a period of our marriage we now refer to as The Troubles, in the endless Northern Irish civil-conflict sense of the phrase.

Looking back, I could cast myself as a sort of innocent Nancy Kerrigan: playing by the rules, playing my role, never guessing that I was about to be smashed in the knee by a real-life Tonya I'll call . . . Tami.

Tami—in a truly Tonya-like detail of this story—was married to the guy who cut and foiled my hair. I'll call him Josh. When Josh heard that Rus was making a movie and that the main character was a desperate single mother who had turned to armed robbery, he urged Tami to audition. Josh and Tami were about to split up—they still loved each other, Josh said, but since the kids had come along they fought all the time and just couldn't seem to live together—and he thought this would be a great morale-booster for her. She'd been really supportive of his new band and he wanted to be equally supportive of her creative dream, which was acting.

Rus auditioned at least a dozen women for the role in what he was now calling *Spree*. Tami, with her gritty voice and velvet-brown curls, was the standout.

If you can see where this story is going, you're way ahead of where I was, vision-wise, at the time. It was now the spring of 1994 and my story about a mom who runs away had grown into a messy novel whose main character was a truck stop whore. My plan was to take a road trip to scout some of the locations in my book after Rus was done shooting

Spree. The documentary about African art had long since been abandoned (lots of people thought it was a good idea but no one wanted to fund it), as had much of my low-paying freelance work. We were focused on *Spree*, on Nick and Claire, on my writing, and on making sure Rus did just enough network news shoots to pay the bills.

It still amazes me, sometimes, to think of all the changes we had not simply checked off the list the way young couples do, but run towards, arms open, in our first seven years together. We had started off by quitting our TV news jobs—good jobs in the country's number-twelve market at a time when TV news still had a few shreds of dignity, a little of the old Ed Murrow tradition in the air—to travel around the world for ten months. To us, quitting when we did made all the sense in the world, or at least it made the kind of sense things make when you're in love and the love itself feels so recklessly new, so fresh, that you want all of life to feel that way.

We got married in Scotland and lingered for three months in Europe, staying in pensions with sagging beds and concrete floors so that we could afford to fatten up on tapas and wine and pasta before we started really ripping through our flip-books of Air India tickets: $1500 per person to fly all the way around the world.

We consumed whole new countries eagerly, like kindergartners running out onto new playgrounds: India, Nepal, Thailand, Malaysia, Indonesia, Australia. We stopped to rest in oases like Goa, Koh Samui, and Java, where we could stay cheaply for a few weeks, read and write travel stories, a half dozen of which were published by the *Seattle Times*, including an account of our ragtag wedding in Scotland that was printed on Valentine's Day.

In that pre-email era, it was Mom who sent our story clippings and other forwarded mail to American Express offices around the world. She also managed our bank account. She did these chores for Caroline, too, during Caroline's Peace Corps stint and post–Peace Corps travel. She did it all while teaching full time. And as she began to wonder what was going on with her brain.

We came home flat broke but got snapped up right away for

election-season gigs at our old station. Then—about five minutes after deciding to ditch birth control—I was pregnant. And I was offered a completely different kind of job, doing public relations for the Seattle Art Museum. And we took out a loan to buy an expensive camera so Rus could freelance for the networks.

Three years later, with a second baby on the way, I left the museum job because my salary would have barely covered daycare for two and it just didn't make sense. So I was doing freelance work, both PR and TV, as much as I could manage with my patched-together childcare combo: Rus when he was available, Mom a few days a week with Nick, and pre-school for Claire.

In five years, I'd gone from the frenetic hothouse of a city newsroom to the solitude of being at home with a baby and a toddler. And home was no longer an apartment a mile up Queen Anne Hill from the Space Needle: it was a house in Seward Park, a quiet lakeside neighborhood where there were many old-growth trees and, in the mid-1990s, even fewer cafés or shops than the few we have now. When Rus was in town, life was, mostly, what I had always hoped our life together would be: time to work, time with our children, time with each other, in proportions that yinned and yanged all over the place but usually felt right. When he was out of town, the time to work shrank and the time with Nick and Claire grew, and it was still mostly sweet, though I missed sharing it with Rus. And sometimes of course it wasn't sweet at all; it was exasperating, like life with toddlers just is, and at those times I felt a little crazy, like new mothers just do, especially a new mom like me who happened not to have very many other new-mom friends and whose husband happened to travel a lot on short notice, or no notice. And whose mother was starting to do things like lose her car or forget every-thing you just told her ("Rus is gone for *how many* days?").

The surprise gift in all of this was that the creative writer in me—the writer of stories who had never quite figured out how to co-exist with the TV journalist—saw her opening and grabbed it. There was some-thing about all the physical work and play of solo motherhood that unlatched my creative mind. When you're building a tower of blocks with a one-year-old and knocking it down, over and over again, your mind can go places. You can grab a crayon and make a few notes. When he's sleeping, you can get down a page on the computer.

It's hard to describe how important this felt to me. It was a little like getting your appetite back after seasickness or the flu: that joy of feeling a good, sharp hunger pang and knowing you're going to eat again and it's going to taste *good*. I had been a prolific writer as a little girl. I kept writing as a teenager and college student, even though my confidence was often shaky. I won the fiction prize at Wellesley. Then in my twenties, I just sort of stopped. I blamed work. I blamed my first husband's depression and his cynicism about all things literary after getting turned down by the English Lit PhD program on which he'd staked his future. I also beat up on myself a lot, imagining alternate lives in which I had not married Dick and had not become a TV news writer but instead had been gutsy enough to go live in a garret, support myself waitressing, and become a real writer, producing stories and novels instead of the five-o'clock report.

But now, here I was spending hours per day pushing a stroller, mixing playdough, finger painting, sidewalk-chalking, reading picture books, turning dishtowels into capes and scarves into princess costumes—and sure, part of me missed ripping news stories off the AP teletype but another part of my brain was stirring and stretching and coming out of hibernation.

I needed some guidance and camaraderie, so I started taking evening writing classes at the UW Extension. By the time Rus was getting ready to shoot *Spree*, I was in my third quarter with Rebecca Brown, who was very good at being simultaneously tough and encouraging. My story about the mom who ran away wouldn't stop growing, though it kept changing protagonists: first it was focused on Runaway Mom (who was not unlike me in 1994: college-educated, underemployed, two young kids), then on a thirteen-year-old girl that Runaway Mom picked up hitchhiking (a girl who just happened to be a lot like me at thirteen: shy, dreamy, a bookworm). Then my focus shifted to that girl's mother, who had become a truck stop whore after running away from home at sixteen (back in the seventies when I was sixteen) and had since cleaned up her act and married a truck driver. Rus and I had personally known or known of a few people whose lives had provided some inspiration for my characters, but mostly I had no idea, from one day to the next, where it was all coming from.

I was thirty-seven years old. Claire was four and was already "writing" her own stories and plays and Nick was not quite two and always ready to throw on a cape and be in her shows. It had been nearly seven years since I said yes to Rus in Haiti. We didn't get to work together very often any more, but we loved being parents together and we loved helping each other make our creative dreams come true. I was writing a book. Rus was making a movie. And he had a good cast. We were both sure that Tami would bring *Spree* to life.

I was only able to visit the *Spree* set a few times during the five days of shooting, since my main job was to be with the kids and answer the phone at home. Rus had a cell phone, but it was a 1994 cell phone that weighed about six pounds and had an anemic battery and very little range in hilly Seattle.

I remember arriving at the first location, an abandoned industrial site full of wooden pallets stacked twenty high alongside rows and rows of empty orange oil drums, where Rus was shooting a chase scene. Even though I'd seen the crew list and the shooting script, I remember how startled I was by the bustle of it all: the lights and the cables and the guys in black with all kinds of equipment hanging off their belts. And then I was surprised by the quiet. They were in the middle of a shot. I stayed back, behind them, behind Rus and Lars, the director of photography. Lars's camera was aimed at the nearest stack of pallets.

And then, there was Tami, rounding the corner of the stack, her fake gun pointed right at the camera. Her brown curls dusty. Her eyes dark with armed-robber intensity. There she was, walking right towards the lens, then stopping ten feet shy of it, frozen, as if she were sighting a target.

"Cut!" Rus yelled, and all at once conversation hummed.

I remember feeling very—wholesome. Blue-eyed. Like I was Florence

Henderson and I'd just strolled over from the *Brady Bunch* set. Tami had that power I didn't have, that unstudied sultriness, like she just couldn't help it, like even in dirty sweats she would still be just naturally intriguing, whether she wanted to be or not.

I didn't perceive Tami's look, on that day, as a personal threat.

Indeed, I had no suspicions at all, no idea that, the minute I took off on my week-long, novel-related road trip down I-5 to snoop around towns like Yreka and Red Bluff, she and Rus would fall into bed, acting on the powerful attraction they felt for each other, like so very many green directors and fresh starlets have done before them. No idea. Not for more than a year.

I take that back. I did feel something that I hadn't previously felt from Rus, something I couldn't quite identify. He was—distracted? Of course. This was something he'd never done before. Everyone else on the set had one job; the director had to know and track them all. He was—obsessed? Naturally. This was his lifelong dream, to make a real movie. I was—invisible to him? Yes. But just temporarily, I told myself, while he's doing this all-absorbing thing. Even though I'd never been invisible before. Even though for seven years our love—our particular love, our own humming, sparking mix of lust and friendship and mutual admiration—had felt as certain as gravity, as certain as the very ground itself, unshakeable through the big quakes like childbirth and through all the little daily tremors too. Our love was in the same category of total seismic unshakeability as my Mom's love for me, or my love for Nick and Claire. There was no need, ever, to question it, just no need.

I don't know all the details—the when, where, how many times—of what happened between Rus and Tami. What Rus told me, more than a year later, was that it was an infatuation that went too far. A two-way attraction born of working together intimately and creatively: not unlike what had happened between us at the TV station. He said it was brief, that he ended it, that he thought he'd put it behind him, that it was over, that not telling me was the right thing to do because he would never let it happen again.

He wasn't going to tell me. He had hoped I would never know. As if it made any sense to have secrets from each other.

But then something unexpected happened. A small production company in Los Angeles saw *Spree*, liked it, and wanted to back a feature-length version with the same cast. Could Rus expand the storyline and reassemble the cast and crew in the summer of 1995?

The L.A. people were in such a big hurry that Rus had to finalize the contract while we were up at the Crystal Mountain ski area near Mt. Rainier, spending a weekend with my sister Lisa and her family and Mom, nine of us crammed into a ramshackle condo that the kids loved because it had a loft with triple bunk beds. The weather was icy and the children were all so little they could barely walk on the slick snow, let alone on skis, so we grownups spent a lot of time playing poker while Nick and Claire and their cousins turned their bunks into forts. But Mom kept forgetting the rules ("Now are aces *high* or *low*?") and Rus kept having to answer his six-pound cell phone, shouting contract details to the production company executive, who was in Israel and wanted him to fax back signed pages from the ski area's office to him, in Israel, right away.

This time, the shoot would be ten days instead of five. This time, as we got closer to shooting, the radar signals I was picking up were a little more psychotic. But I thought I was the crazy one. Why was I so needy? Why couldn't I just focus on my writing and on the kids?

Maybe I should get more involved, I thought. Be more supportive. I offered to do publicity. I wrote and faxed press releases and made phone calls, inviting local papers to visit the shoots and interview Rus and Tami. I also agreed to play a small role as a trashy clerk at a convenience store where Tami shoplifts a few items. I had to wear a lot of makeup and a really tight T-shirt in order to make my TV mom self look trashy enough.

But I still felt weirdly invisible to Rus. And, unbelievable though it seems to me now, I still wasn't even close to guessing why.

On the last day of the shoot, I left for the Squaw Valley Writers Conference. I was so excited. It would be an opportunity to get feedback, go to lots of readings, maybe even meet an agent or an editor who might, just might, take a look at my manuscript. I told Rus I was sorry I'd miss the wrap party, but he assured me it was OK.

When I called home from Squaw Valley, Rus didn't seem terribly interested in talking to me, even though I was having a good week and had lots to tell him about the workshops and parties and the agent who liked my first chapter and the famous authors arriving each evening by helicopter. This hurt. I felt like I was boring him. It unnerved me; I wasn't used to it. I scolded myself: All this silly, neurotic *neediness* I was feeling! Rus was being such a good dad while I was gone; so focused on the kids. What was my problem? Besides, as my grandma would have said, being needy is so unattractive: the surest way to drive your man away.

When I got home, Rus let me feel alternately boring and frantic for about a week or so, while he spent his days in an editing room with the screen version of Tami.

Then he told me he wanted to separate.

When he told me, I had just walked in the door after a day-long freelance gig that included a flight into the Mt. St. Helens blast zone.

Later, much later, I got some mileage out of this.

At the time, despite the blips of radar, despite the neediness, hearing him say such a thing truly felt as unexpected and catastrophic as a volcano erupting. But not Mt. St. Helens: this was a volcano that wasn't expected to erupt, at least not in our lifetimes. Mt. Rainier, maybe, suddenly burying Tacoma and Seattle in a highway of hot mud. Mt. Fuji. Mt. Everest. I couldn't even take it in. It was like volcanic lava had just poured through my brain and instantly rendered thinking, as I had previously known it, impossible. Thinking now made me want to throw up. I remember starting to shake all over, like I had a violent, feverish, heroin-addict-style chill, even though it was a warm August night.

First he tried to say it was all about me. I wasn't passionate enough about my writing, for example. Which is the only item I remember clearly from his list of my shortcomings, because it was the one that really stung, coming so soon after the high of Squaw Valley.

But then Tami's name finally came up, and the truth, and the sick realization that while I was off being as passionate about writing as I was able, given that I am more of a Florence Henderson kind of a person than a Tonya Harding or a Tami—meanwhile, back at the ranch, Rus and Tami were busy stoking their passion for each other.

I have to say I am having a hard time, right now, getting passionate about writing the rest of this. But I also know that it's a part of the story I can't just leave out. So I'm going back to my journals for some help, though it feels a little like going back to the part of the blast zone that's best left roped off forever.

"If only I were suicidal," I wrote on August 21, 1995. "Unfortunately, I think I'm stuck with this life I apparently have managed to fuck up beyond belief."

We did separate that summer. It was surreal and horrible. Nick said, years later, that his enduring memory of that time is seeing me cry a lot, even though I thought I was doing so well at not sobbing in front of him and Claire. Maybe what he remembers is hearing me after he and Claire went to bed, and I went downstairs to cry.

We went to marriage counseling and I cried a lot there too and so did Rus. The counselors said it was clear we both cared a lot about each other, even though I threw a water bottle at Rus during one session. They said, and Rus said, that he was the miserable and confused one and that I was the "grounded" one, which made me feel like a reliable electric plug.

By October, Rus was encouraging me to hope, though I was wary. In mid-November, he finally said, I want to come home.

Four days later, I ventured into an actual church one Sunday morning for the first time in twenty years, feeling some of the same mix of hope and wariness around religion that I felt around Rus. Either I was lucky that day, or God was paying attention to my ripped-up life. I had stumbled into a church where the main themes seemed to be open-armed tolerance, unconditional love and that central, most deeply counter-cultural message of all: forgiveness.

Rus vowed that he was over his obsession. He and Tami were done, and I forgave him and believed him and he came home.

But, damn it all, they weren't done.

For a year and a half, we lived in what I thought was sort of a healing, post-Irish-peace-talks kind of happiness. Nick and Claire were thrilled to have things back to normal. And that's how it felt: normal. We were all reveling in re-discovering Normal, which for us meant routines like our old Saturday morning ritual of getting in bed with giant chocolate and poppy-seed muffins and watching cartoons together: it had become our own little four-person, weekly protest against the puritanical healthiness that ruled the world of young families in Seattle and for us it was the epitome of our Normal.

There were some landmines. We had to walk carefully. For example, we used to joke openly about Rus's reputation around the TV station as an artistic prima donna, but that wasn't very funny any more, at least not coming out of my mouth. Just as it wasn't funny if Rus joked about my love of sleeping a good seven or eight hours a night—which at the time was about two or three more hours a night than he was sleeping—since he had recently named this need for sleep as one of my weaknesses.

But being careful required a constant tenderness that kept us aware that we were repairing something important. We were nursing our relationship the way you nurse a child recovering from the flu. We rested a lot. We served each other comfort foods.

I even made Rus a big, corny Valentine's Day collage about how happy I was to have us back together. I photocopied some pages from my journals and cut the copied pages up—I was going for little snippets of ordinary happiness: place names that meant something to us, funny things the kids said—and then I mixed the scraps with red and orange tissue paper torn into heart shapes and glued it all onto cardboard—and this thing was big, poster-sized.

I remember well how big it was, because one night in the summer of 1997, I carried it out to the driveway, set it down, poured lighter fluid all over it, threw a match on it, and watched it burn.

The summer had started off so well. I had an agent who was confident that she would sell my novel. Mom had agreed to some more tests that might help us figure out what, if anything, could be done to help her with her memory problems. Rus and I would soon be celebrating our tenth wedding anniversary. Claire was turning eight and hosting her first big slumber party. Nick was five and in love with Pokémon. I was starting to work on a second novel inspired by my Finnish-immigrant roots.

I was in Minneapolis, spending a precious two days doing research at the Immigrant History Research Center, on my way to New York for a reunion with my best college friends, when Rus told me on the phone that he was losing it again: he didn't think he could stay married, but hey, no hurry—we'd talk about it when I got home from New York.

This time, it was more like being doused by a random shower of toxic space garbage than slammed by an erupting volcano. This time, I described myself in my journal as "sad as a bowl of oatmeal, but with a few dangerous bubbly hot spots," which may not sound great but was a step up the old self-esteem scale from "I wish I was suicidal."

This time, oatmeal-sad or not, I had some fire in me, some of Mom's pluck, her sisu; some hot spots, like the flames that leaped up from that sappy collage.

I flew home from Minneapolis as soon as I could, which was early the next morning. I told Rus there was no way I could just zip off to New York knowing he was about to blow up our marriage again. But I don't know why I thought that I could instantly fix things, because of course I couldn't. What could I do about Rus declaring that he couldn't fight it anymore—he was still obsessed with Tami? If he couldn't fight it, how could I?

Maybe this time I'll leave, I thought. Let him take care of the house all alone. But then I thought of Tami and her children being in our house with Rus.

He moved out a few days after my mom was diagnosed with probable Alzheimer's disease and a few days before my agent called to tell me she was running out of editors to whom she could pitch my novel. Many of them wrote the nicest things about it in their rejection letters, but then they all came down to—No. The agent suggested that I really get going on my second book, and maybe she could sell the second one and *then* the first one.

But I no longer, or not for much longer, had a husband to support my writing. And Mom, we now knew, had Alzheimer's disease, so the days of writing and freelancing with her as my casual babysitter were officially over. I had a new fear: what if I was now unemployable? I had a few friends who were trying to get back into the working world after some time off for motherhood and they were having a hard time. I started job-hunting as fast as I could.

I landed a job at what my family and I now refer to as the Scary PR Firm, though that is not quite fair, historically speaking, since there were many good people there who helped me a lot. Like Dave, the computer guy, who helped me hide how far behind I was technologically until I was able to catch up and hold my own. And Deb and Jackie and Liz and Melissa, the youngsters I worked with whose dark humor kept me going and whose later connections, in their own post-scary-PR-firm lives, helped Rus and me build our post-Troubles filmmaking business.

Because we did, finally, in the fall of 1997, get past the Troubles.

I viewed it then and still view it now as a kind of miracle, though at the time, most of my good friends and family members were very skeptical.

There's a CBS angle to how it ended, just as there was to how it began, with the Tonya Harding newsathon. This time, CBS asked Rus to be part of the first American news crew to visit North Korea in forty years. It would be a long trip, with a stopover in Tokyo and a two- or three-day wait for visas in Beijing.

In my memory, the call where he just pretty much cried for several very expensive minutes came from North Korea, but Rus thinks it might have been Beijing. Maybe I like the idea of that call coming from a country that had been closed to visitors for as long as he and I had been alive.

Either way, the timing was, from my point of view, right before the point of no return. I had gotten a job. I had joined that small, liberal, Presbyterian church where I felt at home. My friends and family had been there for me all summer, taking me for hikes, inviting the kids and me over for dinners. Even Mom, though she was not retaining the details, was always ready with a hug and a glass of wine and an invitation to stick around and watch *West Side Story*. I was ready to face a future without Rus, or at least without him as my husband.

But there was something about that phone call. Something real, something I trusted, something that said, *This* is the Rus you said yes to in Haiti, not the Rus who's been half-there these past few years. In his tears—there weren't a lot of words—I wasn't hearing some Belfast-style armistice love; I was hearing his beating heart. Not "I'm going to try" but "here I am."

It wasn't like he came home right away. I didn't want him to come home right away. I had to be sure. Because I had changed: I felt strong and clear, not grounded like a damn plug but grounded like a tree planted near a good stream, grounded like my Finnish great-grandparents, who staked a homestead claim in Montana when they were well past forty and raised six children there.

Back at the Immigrant History Research Center in Minneapolis, I had read that most of the Finnish settlers got along well with the local tribes. The Native Americans admired the Finns' tradition of always building the sauna first and living in it while they built their house. A good practice, the Native Americans thought, a spiritual practice: to purify the family with fire and hot rocks and steam before settling into what would be their home for a long time.

And thirteen years later, here we are, in our same home, though the house has grown. The basement is no longer a concrete tomb: it is the studio where we edit our documentaries and the TV room where we observe important family holidays such as the post-Thanksgiving Friday all-day film festival, which starts with a breakfast of giant muffins. We can't quite all hang out in our bed anymore, now that Nick and Claire are grown up.

Before we know it, the nest will be empty. Our dream is to sell or rent it out for a year while we reprise our round-the-world trip in time for our twenty-fifth anniversary. I know that some of the places we loved will have changed a lot, but so have we. And so has our understanding of love in general and our love in particular. We now understand that traveling to faraway places is easy. That it cannot compare to the hard work you do not every twenty-five years but every season of your life: like pulling up dandelions and crabgrass in the spring so the butter lettuce and chard will have room to grow. We've learned that smugness is a weed, not a flower. That love thrives in a good loamy mix of gratitude, humility, humor, and constant sharing: of joys, griefs, frustrations, chores, hikes, bottles of wine, the first tender lettuce leaves, the first ripe tomatoes.

Mom tried to describe love once, in a poem we found in the file folder that also contained her will and that un-crumpled list of goals.

The poem is called, "To My Children" and it begins:

> I love you all
> Equally is not the right word.
> How can love be measured out?
> Love is infinite, indefinite, pervasive.
> Reaching out, enveloping.
> Love can warm and it can smother.
> It should set free not shackle.
> Understand not criticize.

She must have sometimes felt smothered and shackled by the marital expectations of the 1950s and sixties. And I know her stifled braininess made her competitive with and critical of her husbands. But by loving each of her children so far beyond merely "equally," she did a fine job of setting us free to love other people, of demonstrating that we are all capable of "infinite, indefinite, pervasive" amounts of love.

But love is like God: it's the hardest thing in the world to try to contain in words. It can't be contained, not really, not fully. Which must be why we writers keep trying. It's the Irish in us, whether we're James Joyce or just another wholesome Finn. We're passionate about our work, which so often is all about getting all of our memories, all of our love, our people, our mothers and babies, to sit down at the same table, and maybe just enjoy a few iced mochas and mazurka bars. Together.

Gero Psych

Dan, the nurse's aide with the braid down his back, is from Great Falls. Dr. Sorensen's family is from Anaconda. Everyone at the Seattle Geropsychiatric Center seems to have a Montana connection, whether or not that means anything to Mom. Could she feel something comforting, something Montanan, in Dan's ropy forearms as he ties her restraints? Does she see the smokestacks of Anaconda in Dr. Sorensen's eyes, as he holds his tiny flashlight up to hers, chattering about how his grandpa was a copper miner, just like her dad? Is there anything left of Montana, somewhere deep inside her, underneath the spring avalanche of tangles, the winter whiteout of plaques?

I hope so. I hope there are bits of Montana stuck in odd places in her brain, places where she can hide out so that she doesn't have to always be where her body is: in this dayroom jammed with wheelchairs full of sagging, ragdoll people like her. People who started out in places like Butte, Montana and lived lives and had jobs and raised children, never knowing that their destination was this River Styx of a wing of a sprawling hospital in sprawling North Seattle, a carelessly built neighborhood at its sodden worst at this darkest, dreariest time of the year, when the Christmas trees lie lifeless on the curbs next to packing boxes disintegrating in the rain in front of ramblers put up in a hurry fifty years ago that look like they too might cave in at any moment.

What has happened to Mom's brain, what brought her to this joyless place, is not unlike what has happened to her Montana hometown. In its prime, Mom's brain balanced teaching junior high English to refugees, raising six children, dating a widower with three kids of his own. In

105

its prime, Butte was laced with firmly planked, interconnecting tunnels humming with human activity, rich with copper ore. Now, Butte is gouged open, scraped clean, dominated by a giant pit full of toxic wastewater that kills every doomed bird that tries to land on its oily surface, just as the plaques and tangles in Mom's brain kill every thought that dares to fly from one neuron to the next. There might be a fluttering of recognition—the taste of chocolate pudding, a daughter's voice, sunlight striping through the blinds—but rarely enough lift-off to form a sound, let alone an airborne word.

The constant misfiring wears her down; when she drops off to sleep her chest goes up and down like an injured robin's. But it also makes her frustrated, furious, and even if she can't string a sentence together, she can get that rage to her muscles. And that is why she's here. Seattle Gero Psych is the fourth world of dementia care, where they take the hopeless, helpless patients that no one else will take: patients who are a danger to others or to themselves.

That would be our mom, on both counts.

A week ago, on her second night in the Fairview Terrace—the shiny new assisted living home that specializes in Alzheimer's care where we had moved her after two years at the Lakeview—Mom had wandered into the wrong room and pushed a tiny, frail woman out of the bed she thought was her own. It was well after midnight. No one saw it happen. But imagine: You have no short-term memory, you're in a place you've never been before, you wake in the night because you have to pee. You grope your way into the bathroom but then coming out, which way is your bed? You turn the wrong way, open a door into a hallway, grope along the wall, find another door and open it. Ah, there's the bed! But when you throw back the covers, you see a gnarled creature older than time, a goblin, a hag, and you scream and push her out as quickly as you can!

And imagine: you are that ancient, mute neighbor and you're shaken from your dementia-draped sleep by a vigorous seventy-year-old and pushed to the floor hard enough to give you a black eye that covers half your face.

Now imagine: you are that ancient woman's adult child and you are enraged, threatening to sue. *How could the Fairview let this happen? There must be consequences!*

Fairview asked us to have a family member stay with Mom around the clock, "until she became oriented." We complied. It was Christmas week. My twenty-one-year-old nephew volunteered for the overnight shifts. On the fifth night, the night before Christmas Eve, Matthew came to relieve his mother, my sister Kristie, and they were standing outside Mom's room for a moment, talking about how she was doing, when she suddenly woke, tried to get out of bed, and hit her forehead on the corner of the bedframe so hard that blood started pouring out.

Mom was panicking and in pain. An ambulance was called. Kristie rode with her to the hospital a few blocks away. Matthew followed by car. By the time they got to the ER, Mom was beside herself with anxiety and terror and refused to lie still while her wound was cleaned. So she was restrained and sedated and the next thing we knew, we were being told that she needed a stint in Gero Psych, that she wasn't ready to go back to her new assisted living home—the one we'd searched so hard for, that specialized in Alzheimer's care, that promised us everything was going to be OK, that even had a director from Butte, Montana who knew Mom was going to love it there.

You hear "sedation" and you think rest and relief. But because the ER staff believed she was hallucinating, Mom was given Haldol, an anti-psychotic medication that can take weeks to wear off. Before Haldol, she was walking and, albeit often illogically, talking. After Haldol, her body literally curled into a stiff gnome-shape that had to be lifted in and out of wheelchairs. Her gaze turned glassy. She mumbled gibberish. She drooled.

At Seattle Gero Psych, as the Haldol slowly worked its way out of her system, she began to flail and yell and rage. Dan, from Great Falls, tried not to restrain her any more than was necessary.

I remember a friend telling me that all she knew is that she could never put her father in a nursing home. I remember sitting with Mom at Seattle Gero Psych, spooning yogurt into her mouth, thinking, Easy for her to say. Easy for anyone to say who has never been *here*. Never been surrounded by these anguished, thrashing, moaning, babbling faces. Never seen dementia at its torturous, devil-incarnate worst.

I wanted to leap up and go get that friend and bring her back to Gero Psych with me. Make her plead with my mom to eat, just a little, please, Mom, you'll feel better if you eat a little! Make her try to gently uncurl Mom's stiff limbs. Make her hum a tune that might be soothing while she stroked Mom's knotted brow: *Hush, little baby, don't say a word.*

I remember scolding myself, reminding myself that we were all very tired: not just me and my family members and all the people at Seattle Gero Psych, but the whole country, including my friend. It was January 2002. We were not yet accustomed to being a nation at war. 9/11 still felt like yesterday. My brother, who lived in a commuter town in New Jersey that had suffered its share of 9/11 losses, mostly young fathers just like him, was having trouble sleeping or eating. No one I knew, on either coast or in between, was sleeping well.

My last really good sleep had been in the very early morning hours of September eleventh. In my dream, I was strolling through Pompeii and it was so gently breezy and lush, so quiet after noisy Naples, that I didn't want to wake up; I wanted time to stop like it had in Pompeii. But the alarm rang and I went downstairs to make my children's lunches, and I turned on the radio and you know the rest.

I really did visit Pompeii when I was nineteen and it was indeed peaceful. Walking the grassy lanes, looking into the windows of all the carefully excavated homes where everything had ended in an instant, I remember being moved not so much by the implied terror of that last moment but by the evidence of simple pleasures, the glimpses of the lives the Pompeians had lived: bread baking in the oven, wine in the press, a puppy under the table. They had lived two thousand years ago, but they were not so different from me, a college girl seeing ancient places for the first time. They had boisterous families like my own tribe back in green, volcanic Seattle. They loved each other and made meals together. They listened to music and put art on their walls.

I don't know why I dreamed of Pompeii, twenty-five years later, on that night of all nights. We'd had an earthquake in Seattle back in February 2001, and I had crouched in a doorway and watched the kitchen sway back and forth, crockery smashing to the floor. Maybe the quake was on my mind.

Mom had not noticed that February earthquake, even though the epicenter was very near her retirement home. My sisters and I were alarmed by this. Surely it was a sign that her downhill slide was accelerating. An earthquake is something you physically feel, that stays with you, viscerally, for a long time. She had also not really taken in the fact that we had a new president, one that should have outraged her after her many decades as an enthusiastic Democrat.

But by September eleventh, we were way beyond wondering about her awareness of political or seismic events. She had stopped bathing, shampooing, or washing her clothes. She would not let the staff in to clean her apartment. She resisted our help, too, though Kristie got pretty good at getting her clothes laundered and her piles of shoes, CDs, and magazines sorted. Lisa scooped up the mail and bills and Caroline took her to the supermarket. I got her out for walks on Lake Washington and James, back in New Jersey, managed the modest nest egg that paid her rent. We knew we had to move her to a home that specialized in Alzheimer's care and we were frantically shopping for one.

Fall 2001 was a season when time itself seemed to alternate between inertia and mania, the clock racing as we searched for a new place for Mom, driving all over Seattle, listening obsessively to NPR—the frantic search for bodies at Ground Zero, the constant drumbeat to war—and then the clock nearly stopping when we spent time with Mom, trying not to help as she doggedly put on her shoes, trying to look interested as she said the same thing over and over.

Inertia and mania had come to define my work life, too. I had been hired to do media trainings for a coalition of grassroots environmental organizations all over the Rocky Mountain West. The idea was to get ranchers, farmers—the people who lived in all the places the Bush administration was proposing to open up to gas and oil drilling—comfortable with telling their stories. It was a tough schedule—eight Saturdays, with

Saturday stayover flights to make it affordable for the nonprofits who were paying the bill—which for me would mean not only burdening my sisters with more Mom care but missing all those weekends with my children, then nine and twelve. Though I hadn't done a lot of this kind of work, my colleagues thought I was the right one for the job, so I was trying to have faith in their faith in me. "Just be yourself," they said. "Talk about your news experience and your family's Montana roots and Rus coaching Nick's basketball team and they'll love you."

The first training was supposed to take place in western Colorado on September fourteenth. We put it off for a week.

Walking into the sluggish chaos of Sea-Tac Airport on September twenty-first, I saw what this assignment would now be, now that the world had changed: hours of airport and airplane inertia draped in trembling dread, followed by the mania of leading an eight-hour training, followed by more dread-soaked inertia on the trip home. All of it infused with longing to just be with my family, with sorrow that Mom was slipping away, with guilt that I wasn't doing my share because I'd said yes to this crazy job. And yet the work felt more important than ever. "Conservation is patriotic," I kept telling first myself and Rus and later the people who came to the trainings. "If we rip open the Rockies for a few drops of oil and gas, the terrorists win."

So while my mom searched for shoes and stashed her dirty underwear in the kitchen cupboard and her shampoo in the refrigerator and her CDs in the VCR, I spent my weekends flying and driving through the landscape that had shaped her—a world where everything, to my Seattle eyes, was vividly, sharply drawn: the sun setting hard and quick behind zig-zagging peaks, the morning main streets of Durango or Trinidad or Billings or Great Falls as harshly shadowed as Edward Hopper's diners and hotel rooms. Mom had been an artist, too, though she preferred to paint from photos she took on her travels. Maybe the deep contrasts of sunny places like Greece and Italy suited her Montanan eye better than the soft grays outside her Seattle window. She was still painting, occasionally, with an artist friend of ours; her most recent works resembled my three-year-old niece's.

The Saturday trainings humbled me. I may have been tired all fall, but many of the people who came to the trainings were near collapse. On top of running their ranches and farms and businesses, they were fighting sudden and aggressive bureaucratic nightmares: drilling had begun on land they'd leased to graze their cattle for generations, or under their child's school, or next door to the home they'd sold their city house to buy, the home where they dreamed they'd start a new life. They could barely afford to give up a Saturday, and yet they came. They wanted to learn how to tell their stories. They wanted to believe that reporters could help them. Some of them had just found out that the mineral rights on their own land were not in fact their own, and drilling was about to begin. Some had just learned that drilling was already under way, deep below their neighborhood, and that's why toxic plumes were occasionally flaring up out of the storm drains. Others had just learned that the land their grassroots group had been struggling to protect, or their tribe's sacred burial place, or their county park, was now officially open for gas and oil exploration. For them, the war on terror was not taking place in some faraway country; it was happening on their own back forty. They'd been to places like Butte, Montana: they knew what the future could look like.

Nine years later, the Bush era is finally over and I wonder how they're all doing. I haven't kept up. I could blame the frenzied, fall 2001 pace of the dementia drilling into Mom's brain, which led me to seek work that did not demand so much travel. I know they won a few victories and lost a lot more; I know that the Iraq War sucked media attention away from their struggles, just as it sucked attention away from the gutting of medical research into illnesses like Alzheimer's and hundreds of other quietly committed burglaries during the Bush years.

I know that some of what the Saturday trainees feared was what had happened to Mom. All along the spine of the Rockies, in every town where hard mineral mining and coal, oil, and gas exploration were starting to boom again, there were whispers about cancer clusters and spikes in childhood asthma and unexplained high rates of Parkinson's, multiple sclerosis, ALS and—always in the background, always harder to detect—Alzheimer's disease.

The easy retort to the health whisperers is to say, Every place in our world is toxic. Even deserted islands and Arctic ice floes are drenched in acid rain. We need jobs, we need oil; we can't have either without risk. But some of those stories Mom used to tell over and over again haunt me now. *Nothing grew in Butte. When I was a child, no one even tried to grow grass or trees or flowers in the soil of the Richest Hill on Earth, so my sister and I played in the dirt. We filled old coffee cans with dirt and stirred in water and made mud pies. And the sky was filled with dirt, too: soot and smoke bellowing from the mines, twenty-four hours a day.*

Nothing green may have grown, yet Mom grew just fine. Early on, she was pegged as a high-achieving girl, a girl whose brain was something special.

Now, in the fall of 2001, as the world reeled and recoiled and tried to right itself after 9/11, my mom's brain was reeling too, finally buckling under the long assault of plaques and tangles.

Alzheimer's disease does not progress in a smooth, downward line. My sisters and I knew this. But the steep slope she was on that autumn caught us all by surprise. In hindsight, we can see clearly that we missed our chance to move her when she might have been able to weather it better. And we can see that our first mistake had been to move her, in 1999, from her house to the one retirement home she deemed acceptable, thanks to its view of Lake Washington—even though it did not have an Alzheimer's wing—because we wanted so badly to believe she could stay there for a while before we'd have to move her again.

But she was there only two years before we saw that the time had come.

So we frantically looked and finally found the Fairview Terrace, and Sheila from Butte assured us it was all going to work out just fine. On a December afternoon we orchestrated the move. Caroline took Mom home to her house for the day while the rest of us packed and moved and unpacked her belongings. She was moving from a one-bedroom apartment to one room. We had a few weeks to clean out the Lakeview apartment, so we focused on making her new room look familiar: putting her paintings and photos on the walls and her afghan on the bed.

Fairview was decorated for Christmas and it felt festive. We reasoned that it was a good time to move because the Christmas celebrations at the Fairview and at our homes would be a good distraction for Mom.

Just the day before moving day, I had taken her to see the Christmas pageant at our church, featuring a motley band of kids dressed up in towels and sheets, including our daughter Claire as an angel and our son Nick as a shepherd. Getting her up and clothed and making it to church on time had been a sweaty ordeal and I was embarrassed by her awful, greasy hair and ashamed of myself for being embarrassed and also ashamed for wishing I could just relax and enjoy the pageant without worrying about whether Mom might shout out something strange in the middle of a quiet moment. But we made it and she saved her shouting for the Christmas carols, which she belted out with gusto.

I wish I'd known that the pageant would be the last grandchildren's event she would ever attend—the last public event, period. I wish I had simply savored the fact that she was there instead of brooding about her hair and whether there was any way to persuade her to let one of us wash it. I wish I'd known that this homespun pageant was as close to Christmas as Mom was going to get that year, or any year for the rest of her life.

But of course I didn't know, I couldn't know, that she would live at Fairview Terrace for exactly five days. That she would push an old woman out of bed and then, a few nights later, crack her head open getting out of her own bed. That she would spend Christmas in the hospital in a Haldol fog and be discharged to a place we'd never heard of called the Seattle Geropsychiatric Center, better known as Gero Psych. That before 2001 became 2002, we'd see our Mom in restraints, because although she was now unable to hold a spoon, she was still strong enough to hit and hurt the Gero Psych nurses and aides.

The hardest part of the Christmas pageant had not been Mom's greasy hair or worrying about what she might do. The hardest part had been seeing the other grandmas, well-coiffed, in dry-cleaned holiday sweaters, gently smiling, tearing up when their own grandchildren bravely shouted out their lines. Sitting in the Gero Psych day room ten days later, coaxing Mom to eat some yogurt, it was thinking about those grandmas that made me want to cry. Or rage.

The fourth world. When people said that about countries like Haiti, they meant that it was hopeless. And that was what was going on at Seattle Gero Psych. Patients and their families were being purged of hope. Taught how to live without it, because there really wouldn't be any more. It was a hard lesson to learn. I can imagine, that for Dan and Dr. Sorensen and the others, it was also hard and heartbreaking to teach. For eight Saturdays in the Rocky Mountains that fall, I had been trying to teach people to hold on to hope in the worst of circumstances, not knowing that at the end of the season I would have to accept that there was no more hope for Mom. No more pageants, no more walks, no more joy.

John the Divine

When people ask about Mom's Alzheimer's disease and what it was like for me and my brothers and sisters, I don't talk a lot about John, partly because he was not around much during the last decade of her life and partly because it—he—was so complicated. My big brother wanted so badly to remain part of our family. But John couldn't seem to stop himself from sabotaging one dinner, one Christmas, one family relationship after another.

He was my mother's first born and his brain, like hers, was strangled to death—though the strangler was not Alzheimer's, it was a brain tumor, and it moved like a serial killer, skilled and quick. Five weeks. But long before his dramatic and early exit on a leaky winter day in 2004, John stood apart, marked, a prophet.

He looked like Jesus and he raged like Jeremiah. As a young man, he was John the Baptist, urging us all—from Mom down to four-year-old Caroline—to take the plunge into a new, anti-establishment world order of peace, love, marijuana, LSD, personal computing, alpine skiing, and free long-distance phone calls courtesy of a gizmo known as the Black Box. He was John the Evangelist, exhorting us to listen to his revelations of the end of time, the many layers of space, the several kinds of infinity. He was Jonah, spewed out by the whale, stumbling through Nineveh, sounding his lonely alarm: Only forty days, citizens! This decadent, cocktail-party culture is doomed!

But it wasn't Nineveh that had only forty days; it was John.

He would tell you, if he could, that he was marked for struggle before he was born, because the first thought anyone ever had of him was:

Mistake. Not wanted. My mother would tell you, if she could, that once she knew she was pregnant, at nineteen, of course John was wanted. That she and her young fiancé accepted the call. They got married. They found a tiny home to shelter their newborn child. John's father pursued his trade: he enrolled in dental school. His mother, our mother, gave up her own dreams to support her husband and care for her new baby.

Their first home was an apartment in an old brick building, long gone now, torn down for the 1962 World's Fair. The Seattle Rep's oddly curved Bagley Wright Theatre stands where it once stood.

Their second home was another apartment in another brick building, a little California-style, courtyard cluster in north Seattle. That was where John's dad told Mom he was leaving her and John and baby Kristie for their close mutual friend Connie and for Paris—France, not Texas—where, unbelievably, he was posted during the Korean war: a freshly minted dentist to the troops.

Fifty years later, in February of 2004, I had tickets—purchased weeks before the brain tumor—to see the Rep's production of William Saroyan's *The Time of Your Life* with John's ex-wife Rebecca and two of his sons. We had a mutual friend in the cast. As the show date approached, we decided we would still go. It would be a break in the tension of keeping vigil at John's bedside; our other brother and sisters and John's father would all be there with him. But at the last minute, Rebecca cancelled. She had a hunch that this rainy Sunday would be the day of John's death, she later said, and she was right.

Who knows? Maybe John was more able to time his last breath than we ever could have guessed. He waited until his sons were by his side. He waited until some of the rest of us were seated over the site of his first home, watching a drama about the brevity and poignancy of life. And, like an Old Testament numerologist, he waited for the most mathematically supple date at hand: Leap Year Day, February 29, 2004.

"In the time of your life, live—so that in that wondrous time you shall not add to the misery and sorrow of the world, but shall smile to the infinite delight and mystery of it," Saroyan wrote. The poignancy of his prose, the empathy with which he sketched his quintessentially

116

American cast of barroom dreamers! And yet, according to the Rep's program notes, the playwright himself was "passionate and arrogant," a man who had "little use for the niceties of society, and frequently rubbed people wrong with his outspoken opinions and fiercely held principles." Saroyan was a man like my brother, who longed to "smile to the infinite delight and mystery of [life]," but knew that much as he longed to, he simply couldn't.

John comes back to me now, after death, my memories of him transformed into images of prophesy, crucifixion, annunciation, ascension.

When our big family gathers for Christmas, drinks clinking, hors d'oeuvres passing, I see him circa 1970, a bone-thin college student, on the night he stormed into the stately living room of my paternal grandparents' home and turned over their vast, perfectly polished coffee table, sending glasses crashing and canapés crushing underfoot, raging about materialism, capitalism, imperialism, damning all present with charges of idolatry, hypocrisy, greed, and complacence.

When I lie flat on my back in the night, unable to sleep, I see him, spread eagled on his waterbed, arms outstretched, his Jesus hair fanning out on the pillow, naked except for his white briefs.

Walking into Benaroya Hall to see the Seattle Symphony one wet night the summer before he died, I see him middle-aged but still bursting with urgency, boyishly happy that I have accepted his invitation, lit from behind by the tall rain-streaked windows, launching into a torrential soliloquy about all the stories he wants to tell, whole novels and books, if only he had time to write them down.

Pausing to admire Mt. Rainier on a clear day, I always look just to the left, where there's a kneeling outcrop of the mountain near the ski area we often went to when we were children, John flying down the slopes like a crazy angel while the rest of us, happy but earthbound, gamely snowplowed and stemmed.

Opening my laptop, I think of one day in the early seventies when we stood in the kitchen, arguing about computers—he, home for the summer from M.I.T., me, a dreamy teenager who still wrote in her journal with a fountain pen.

"Someday, Ann, every desk in the world will have a computer on it, even yours!" he yelled and I yelled back that just because he was obsessed, that didn't mean that the whole world was and that I for one would never ever want or need such a thing. Never! Who did he think he was, predicting the future with such confidence?

John wanted what human beings want—love and meaning—but he wanted divinity too. He wanted everyone to see and worship his special flame. He wanted everyone to comprehend that the computer technology he was working on was going to change the world. And from us, his parents and brother and sisters, he wanted even more: he wanted us to recognize his brokenness, to mourn with him for all that had gone wrong in his childhood, to appreciate the hardships he'd suffered, the sacrifices he'd made, as the oldest child in a messy, twice-divorced family. He wanted me, especially, the doted-on firstborn of the "new" family, to feel some measure of his anguish. When we were children, he kept up a constant stream of cruel teasing: *you're ugly, you're spoiled, no boy will ever look at you, why can't you be like your sisters.*

His timing was forever off. Just as he'd been the combustible teenager when the rest of us were cute kids, he was already a scorched, damaged, disillusioned adult when the rest of us were barely launching our post-college lives and beginning to wonder what was up with Mom. With each passing year, John got more angry and more needy and anything any one of us tried to say or do was never enough or never right or just made things worse. Finally, right around the time that Alzheimer's disease was ramping up its sticky assault on Mom's brain, John took his wife and three sons and pulled out of the family altogether.

We missed them. Mom grieved. But John had worn us out. He had worn us down. So we turned away. We had our romances, marriages, jobs, babies; we wanted to live in the wondrous time of our lives. And we wanted to help Mom savor what time, wondrous or not, she still had.

Years passed. Kristie kept in touch with him; occasionally I would hear from him. He had read another book about how feminism had destroyed civilization; if only we would read it, we would understand everything. Or he had finally figured his life out: it was his stepdad, my dad, who was to blame for screwing him up, not his real dad. No, scratch that—it was Mom. Everything was her fault; why couldn't we see that? If she could just apologize, John could forgive her and move on.

When we pointed out that Mom could barely speak at all any more, let alone apologize to him, he was dismissive, as if Alzheimer's disease was a ruse she had cooked up to avoid him. He had not seen her since she moved out of her house. He did not know that she had long ago signed documents giving all of us except for him the power to make her legal, financial, and health care decisions.

A year before he died, though of course we didn't know that at the time, John called Kristie and me, begging for sympathy, after Rebecca told him she wanted a divorce. We were wary. We had already talked to Rebecca and had started the slow process of getting to know her and the boys again.

John was so steeped in his own anguish that he didn't seem to understand when we tried to tell him how far Mom had fallen into the mire of her illness.

Then he started getting such bad headaches that he wondered if it could be the beginning of Alzheimer's. Leave it to John, we said to each other, to turn Mom's illness into an excuse for his own special brand of hypochondria.

And then once again, he was maddeningly right: his brain *was* under siege. And the time of his life was suddenly—gone.

When John was a boy, he focused all of his anger—about his dad leaving, about my dad arriving—on me, the first child of his mom's new marriage. He singled me out for vicious tirades in front of my sisters and urged them to shun me too. But it was never enough. He couldn't stop. He couldn't stop hating. So I hated him back, even though I didn't want to, because I also loved him. I loved him worshipfully, the way little sisters do, no matter how they're treated: he was my big brother, he knew everything, he could do anything, he was smarter and more fascinating than anybody else's big brother.

I longed for him to decide that I was as worthy of his affection as my sisters were. I asked myself, night after night, why I couldn't just stop hating him *or* loving him. Just stop. It wasn't my fault his dad went away. It wasn't my fault that I was his stepdad's first born; I couldn't change that. Why couldn't he forgive me? He looked like Jesus; why couldn't he be like Jesus?

He grew up and, briefly, tried. I can't remember how it started, exactly, but we became tentative friends. I know it was after he left for M.I.T. Maybe when he was home during the summer he caught me poring over his stash of college catalogues. Maybe he could see how badly I, like him, needed to get out of Seattle—which, in 1974, was still mainly known to the rest of the country as the setting for the TV show, *Here Come the Brides*. I was not a math geek like him, but I was an oddball like him, a bookworm and a writer trapped in a town where skiing and boating skills were far more highly valued. He encouraged me to apply to east coast schools, explaining that they were all hungry for "geographically diverse" kids and that I was sure to get financial aid. He was right.

At the end of my freshman year at Wellesley, when he was in graduate school at Berkeley, I called him and told him I wanted to fly to San Francisco and then take the Greyhound Bus home and could I stay with him for a few nights? He said yes and I felt elated and brave and so proud of myself for making the call. I spent a weekend with him and fell in love with the entire state of California, which I had never seen before and which seemed, after my long, homesick year in New England, like an Eden overflowing with sun and tomatoes and strawberries and bare arms and legs and bongo drums. Driving through the Berkeley hills in John's VW bus, sharing joints, I felt like I finally had a big brother, the real kind, the kind you could go to if your parents pissed you off or your boyfriend dumped you.

Half a dozen years later, after I graduated, I became the first member of the family, after John, to have a computer on my desk at work: it was called the NewsStar and it had a squat black screen with orange Courier type. On it, I wrote "rip and read" roundups of wire service news stories for radio stations. Once my editor gave me the go-ahead, all I had to do was press a button and off my roundups went to hundreds of teletypes in hundreds of radio newsrooms. Imagine!

My big brother had imagined.

By the time I was tapping away on the NewsStar, John was well into his career in Silicon Valley, imagining all kinds of things. His first marriage hadn't gone so well but he was absorbed in his work. Then he met Rebecca, a planner for a small city, a skier and an intellectual who could ski and think as fast as he could. They got married and moved back to Seattle. Mom was thrilled. We were all thrilled: we loved Rebecca. We dared to hope that maybe—living with Rebecca, living next door to the mountains he had missed so much—maybe John would be happy, or at least some John-version of happy.

John and Rebecca found a house in a suburb a half hour from the ski slopes. They found good jobs. They had three sons, all bright and beautiful.

But then, somehow, that old anger started to burble up again. Soon Mom, John's dad, my dad, Kristie, me, and eventually Rebecca and the boys were on the firing line.

And then, like Jesus, he suddenly died and set them free. Set us all free.

And now we all have computers on our desks, or in our backpacks. And so John is everywhere.

Early in his career, he worked on something to do with getting computers to produce colors, so I think of him sometimes when I'm shuffling through photos or video. Then he worked on something to do with calendar code, so I think of him when I buy a plane ticket.

It's been six years now since that Leap Year day of my big brother's death. I try to stay in touch with his sons. The oldest is in Chicago, getting a PhD in math. The middle son is studying economics. The youngest is at St. John's College, where they read all the Great Books. John would be proud.

John's oncologist told me she'd been seeing a spike in brain cancers like his among people his age who had worked around computers all of their adult lives. She thought it might be the PVC—all that plastic that houses everything, not the metals and toxins you might suspect.

A few days after his death, I wrote this in my journal: "John believed so wholly in the promise, the force for good, that computers might someday be. And yet they may have killed him. What would he say, from where he is now? Was it worth it, worth a third or more of his potential span of life on this planet? Would he say it was random: Ann, I just drew the unlucky card? Or would he say it wasn't just the PVC plastic off-gassing, it was the stress of being John, of never quite getting how to be smarter than just about everybody and still get along in this world?"

I don't pretend to know where John is or whether his spirit has ever bumped into Mom's or whether he might finally be getting down to resolving his unfinished business with God: finding out why he was called to restless prophecy; why his childhood anger never abated; why the love of his mother, sisters, brother, wife, and sons was never enough; why the time of his life ran out before he could resolve any of that here on planet Earth.

He gave me my first tastes of cruelty and of charisma. He terrified me and he mesmerized me: his intellect was so dazzling; his personality was so damaged, so corroded by the burning anger he felt at such a young age and never knew how to safely cool.

Our lives are far more peaceful without him.

But there's a hole: an odd quiet where there used to be a constant clatter—the kind of clatter, like the old newsroom teletype machine, that could sometimes drive you crazy, especially when you were trying to think.

Then one day the noise is suddenly gone, and you realize, too late, that it was one of the sounds that made you feel truly alive.

If, If, If

"All would be well if, if, if,
Say the green bells of Cardiff . . ."

The question we try not to allow ourselves, we grievers, is the big *What If*. What if Buddy Holly hadn't gotten on that plane? What if my daughter's friend Phaedra had been in her mother's car instead of her aunt's that one summer night when Phaedra had just turned seven, that Texas night when a young drunk driver slammed into the back seat where Phaedra sat and the car burst into flames? What if my mother's brain had not flipped some chemical switch two or three decades before her death; what if that fatal rerouting of proteins into plaques and tangles had never happened? And was it a switch that flipped in a moment, a fateful moment when stress hormones and genes and brain chemistry all crashed into each other just like Phaedra's aunt and the man who'd had a few too many? Or was it a switch that had been rusting and fraying all her life until it finally just couldn't hold on? What if she hadn't played in the Butte dirt as a child and then put her chubby baby hands in her mouth, over and over again?

If, if, if, say the green bells of Cardiff in the old Welsh poem by Idris Davies. Pete Seeger and Judy Collins and the Byrds all recorded versions of it; I can hear their sweet voices and I can hear the bells from all the towns they sang about but the only line I remember is *If, if, if* ringing out over the roofs of Cardiff, a city neither my mother nor I ever visited but one where she might have felt some kinship: the mountains, the mines, the terrible cruel beauty of a landscape that asks a high price to feed a family. Send me your young men and I will turn them old

123

and bent. Give me your offerings of coal and minerals and I will fill the sky with smoke and kill every green thing on the ground and your babies' blood will run with my chemicals. And *if, if, if* you can get away from here, I know where you'll go: to some town in America like Butte, Montana, where the mountains are even higher and the mines are even deeper. And you'll meet miners from all over the world, from Wales and Finland and Sicily and Kentucky, and together you'll go down every day while your wives will raise your children in the dirt and soot spewed out by your smokestacks.

So where do I even start saying *if, if, if*?

What if Mom had not been born in Butte? What if there had been no Great Depression and Grandpa had made more money and it hadn't taken him until Mom was thirteen to move his girls away from the dirty mines and down to the Flats?

No. If I am going to indulge myself in this game of What If, I don't want to go backwards. I want to imagine her as she would be now. Alive. Without Alzheimer's disease.

There's a part of me that wishes I could get her blessing before I go into this imaginary world. There's a part of me that knows what she might say: Oh, honey, don't do it. You've got a beautiful life, you've got Rus and Claire and Nick, why do you want to torture yourself like this? Go out and do something fun with your family! But there's another part of me that wants to do it, for her. To show her, wherever she now is, what might have been. I don't know where she is. I feel her with me, now and then, though I don't know what that even means or how to describe it. But I need her—that Mom that I feel with me, in me, near me—I need her to know that I'm writing this book because I want everyone who reads it to shoulder just for a moment the loss of *her* and then to feel the full weight of that loss times twenty-six million. Twenty-six million people around the world who are slipping away instead of living the lives they could have lived.

What if, instead of caring for them, we could cure them? What if we could keep Alzheimer's from happening in the first place?

What if.

What if she and I were walking in Seward Park right now, instead of me sitting here at my desk looking out at the park and thinking about her? What if her body was still strong, ready to walk, instead of gone? What if I could hear her voice, put my arm around her, bask in her present self instead of her spirit slipping away from me like one of those low clouds weaving through the trees on a wet day that you can see and even walk right through but never ever touch? What if she and I were walking on the path that goes right through the heart of the woods, the oldest trees in Seattle, and we were just breathing in all that fresh tree-air and talking about nothing and everything? Which of the fourteen grandchildren look the most like her. What a beautiful place we live in. What she's going to paint next or where she's going to travel next or which grandchild will be the next to spend the night at her house. What if Mom was seventy-nine years old and alive and that's what we were doing today, right now, and I was writing a book about anything, anything at all besides my mother dying of Alzheimer's disease?

If Mom had not had Alzheimer's disease, her teaching career would have gathered strength and momentum instead of wobbling and sputtering just when she'd finally landed the job she'd always wanted. She might have kept on teaching for ten more years. One hundred fifty students each semester, times twenty. Three thousand students that never got a chance to learn from her.

If Mom had not had Alzheimer's disease, she might have stayed in her airy house in Madrona. I think she'd like the ways the neighborhood has changed. There are more cafés now. She and I could have met at Verité and shared one of its famous cupcakes. I could have introduced her to some of the middle-schoolers at Madrona K–8 School, where I've been volunteering as a writing coach. The old building has been renovated and the principal has won awards for raising test scores, though most of the white kids in the neighborhood still go to private or Catholic schools. Maybe she could have become a Madrona School booster. Worked the Tennis Club crowd. Worn a Madrona K–8 Panther Pride T-shirt on her walks down to the lake through the neighborhood's tonier side. Madrona's school color is sky blue: perfect for Mom with her blue eyes and silver hair.

I wish I could bring her in tomorrow for show and tell. Have her recite that poem she used to love so much by the young Englishman who was about to be executed for treason: "My glass is full, and now my glass is run;/And now I live, and now my life is done." How it used to make me cry, the thought of dying young!

Because of course that's what tragedy is: dying young. You get that look from people, when you use the word "tragedy" to describe Alzheimer's disease: that look that says, Don't say it's tragic. Childhood cancer, that's tragic. Phaedra killed by a drunk driver at seven: tragic. Buddy Holly dead at twenty-two. Chidiock Tichborne, one-hit-wonder poet of the sixteenth century, dead at twenty-eight. Young soldiers killed in senseless wars. Babies dying of malnutrition. Those are tragedies. Not Alzheimer's disease.

But how do we measure tragedy? How do we compare heartbreaks? When a life is slowly, torturously erased instead of suddenly cut short, shouldn't we grieve that loss too? And when this gradual erasure is happening to millions of people, should we not call it what it is: an epidemic?

Every day, I get an email digest called the *Alzheimer's Daily News*. My sisters think I'm a glutton for punishment. But I want to be among the first to know when the really big breakthrough occurs. I want to be first in line for the vaccine trials. I want to read the stories of the first people cured. I want to hear the news when scientists finally figure out which cocktails of genes, environment, stress, and bad luck are most likely to cause Alzheimer's disease and which cocktails of vitamins, nutrition, drugs, mental and physical exercise might prevent it or slow it down. I want to celebrate when brave people with Alzheimer's testify before Congress about the costs of the illness—in lost human potential; lost wages; lost caregivers' wages; in endstage, round-the-clock nursing; in the emotional and social toll on families. I want to mourn when lives, famous and not, succumb to this slowest and most callous of killers.

"Memories Exist Even When Forgotten, Study Suggests," was the headline on an *Alzheimer's Daily News* story I saw today. Scientists using functional magnetic resonance imaging tracked patterns in the brains of subjects that showed that even when the person could not remember the details of a task performed earlier, "the brain knew something about what had occurred, even though the subject was not aware of the information," according to lead researcher Jeff Johnson of the University of California at Irvine.

For a fleeting, absurd moment when I saw that headline, I thought of all of Mom's memories, so many of them gone forever before she could share them and I wondered, Are they *somewhere?* Could they someday be unlocked? But this was a science story, not science fiction, and of course Mr. Johnson was talking about the memories of living people. Young people, in fact: his subjects were college students.

So here comes the big What If again, this time past tense. What If scientists had found a way for Mom to reclaim all those memories she was shedding like snakeskins every day for the last decade or more of her life?

I picture them like boxes of old photographs and letters no one can get to because they're behind or underneath other, heavier boxes, or because they're buried in silt and sludge, like a box that had the bad luck to be stored away in a New Orleans garage when the levees broke.

That's what Alzheimer's disease is like: it's like the levee breaking in your brain, the levee that keeps out the sludgy plaques and seaweedy tangles. Only it happens slowly, instead of all at once like Hurricane Katrina. It happens as slowly as molasses dripping from a cracked jar way in the back of the cupboard. And no one notices until every other jar on the shelf is stuck in it, unable to move, unable to do what it is there to do: to be lifted out easily, to pour out a few drops of oil or a shake of cinnamon or a teaspoon of baking powder and then to be put away again, at the ready, until the next time it is needed to make something tasty and beautiful.

To be put away where it exists, even if forgotten.

I have a few framed photos of Mom in my office. Some came from my Grandma's boxes, including one of Mom and Aunt Jo Ann when they were about four and two. In the photo they are smiling so sweetly, as if they've just heard a silly joke or been promised a gingersnap and that's all it took to capture this radiant little instant in their tiny lives. But if you look closely, you can see the hours of preparation that went into this moment. Their hair is clean and shiny and bobbed just so: the bangs straight across the middle of their foreheads, the ends in perfect half-moons just above their earlobes. Their dresses are lovingly detailed with velvet ribbons and Peter Pan collars and puffed sleeves. Their long stockings are free of rips and holes. Only their scuffed white shoes hint at the sooty Butte world outside. Grandma could cut and shampoo their hair, scrub their faces, sew those beautiful dresses—but she must have run out of steam or spare change for polish when it came to the shoes.

What if I could ask Mom what she remembers about this picture, instead of idly speculating? I know they were very poor then; it would have been the mid-thirties, when they lived in that succession of ever-smaller Finntown flats. It must have been a lot of work to heat water for bathing and shampooing. And the dresses would have had their own whole histories: this one cut from Auntie Helen's castoff, that one from a bolt end spotted in the corner of the Singer store. Aunt Jo Ann's smile is a little tentative; Mom's is trusting, confident. Maybe Mom just told Jo Ann not to worry: Sit still, little sister, fold your hands like mine, smile like I'm smiling, and soon we'll be sent off to play.

Mom would probably tell me that although she knows now how poor they were, she didn't know it then. That her parents and her widowed Finnish grandmothers and her childless Auntie Helen all doted on their two little princesses, all encouraged their game of pretending to be Elizabeth and Margaret Rose of England. I know this from conversations we had decades ago. But what I don't know is what she might say about this picture *now*. She had hoped someday to write about her childhood, to reflect in a way that she never had time for when she was raising six kids and launching a teaching career in the middle of her life.

When we were growing up, she didn't talk a lot about her roots. But as the six of us moved out and her life slowed down to a reasonable speed, she began to take an interest. She regretted that she hadn't learned more from her own parents. Grandpa was the last of his family.

It's breathtaking to think of what we miss by just being in the wrong phase of life at the wrong time. When Grandma and Grandpa were ready to tell their stories, Mom was busy doing everything she could to blend into the Tennis Club crowd. It was the age of assimilation; being ethnic was as uncool then as it is cool now. Mom had a lot going for her in her quest to swim with the Seattle bluebloods: flawless diction, a beautiful smile, a great figure, skin that tanned so deeply and evenly that she joked about being "mistaken for an Indian" and, when pressed, would sometimes say something vague about Finns being "darker" than other Scandinavians—which is not really true, although the Sami people, formerly known as Laplanders, are darker and Mom's coloring probably came from some Sami branch of her genealogy.

But the higher she climbed up the social ladder, the harder it was to climb back down and pull up a chair and sit still while her parents talked. Or Grandpa's sister, dear old Auntie Helen, whose Parkinson's was getting worse and worse. Or Grandma Cere's sisters: Eine, Anna, Laina, and Martha, with their funny Finnish way of saying AR-lene instead of Ar-LENE and their loyalty to the weekly ritual of getting their hair set in unmovable waves and their sudden, late-sixties defection from slippery print dresses to polyester pantsuits in alarming pastels. It was hard to sit still, no matter how much she loved them, especially when her husband and six children were pulling her toward the door, away from the world of the Grundstroms and Warilas and Peltolas and Turppas. And it was probably even harder when her marriage began to splinter and she was scrambling to get a college degree and then a job with six children still clamoring for her attention.

And then, thirty years later, I did the same thing to her.

I was so *busy*. I had children and a marriage and a career and even before we knew it was Alzheimer's, I knew that something was wrong with Mom's brain, I knew her memories were shredding away, going, going, gone, more every day—but maybe some irrational part of me believed that somewhere they *still existed, even if forgotten* by Mom. That when I was ready, I would find them, intact, like boxes in a nice dry basement, as opposed to a post-Katrina New Orleans basement.

It was so hard to sit still for her. I was moving too fast.

Now I'm left with photos that have no stories.

Like my other desktop favorite: a snapshot of Mom teetering between childhood and adolescence, holding a trout in one hand and a fishing pole in the other, her smile a wide, proud beam, her straight hair permed in the tortured style of the early forties, a Girl Scout pin in the middle of her still-flat, T-shirted chest. Was it a Girl Scout outing? Or was she fishing with Grandpa, and just happened to be wearing the pin?

The point is, there's a story and I don't know it. Much as I am grateful for the photo and all that it says, I threw away—like it was nothing at all—the window of time when she could have told the story.

I was so busy.

Twenty years earlier, when I took refuge from the anxieties of high school in our school's ambitious theatre program, my big acting break was landing the role of a mom whose life had not only slowed down, it had ground to a near-halt: Beatrice, the bitter, mentally unstable, divorced mother in Paul Zindel's *The Effect of Gamma Rays on Man-in-the-Moon Marigolds*, who spends most of her stage time in a ragged bathrobe and slippers, smoking and ranting about her "half-life," a phrase she picked up from her daughter's award-winning science experiment in which marigolds were exposed to radiation.

"Half-life. If you want to know what a half-life is, just look at me. You're looking at the original half-life!" I growled as Beatrice, dragging on a Salem. The student teacher had taken me out back behind the art building and taught me how to smoke for the role—it was the seventies—and I was loving it.

Mom had donated her old aqua-blue nylon bathrobe and worn-out slippers for my costume. My long hair was pinned up and purposely straggling from a couple of dozen bobby pins. I penciled crow's feet around my eyes and lines around my mouth.

I wonder now what Mom thought, looking at me up there in her cast-off robe, railing about my wasted half-life, smoking away. Was I acting out her worst nightmare, the version of her story in which she is left alone and falls apart instead of creating a new life?

I think Beatrice was my nightmare, when my kids were young: the nightmare of failure and isolation, the vision that drove me to never slow down.

I look at these pictures of Mom as a girl and I know now: the cost of never slowing down is high. The stories I didn't hear are as gone forever as if they had never existed, as if they were the students Mom didn't teach, the trips she didn't take, the paintings she didn't paint.

Memories Exist, Even When Forgotten. Really? Where?

What if she and I were walking in the park right now and I was listening to her stories?

It is hard to move beyond walking in the park with this whole "What if" line of thinking. Because what she would be in my life, if she were still alive, is such a part of the fabric, the dailiness of it, that it would be impossible to tease out and name the strands: of borrowing things, the way I borrowed her old bathrobe to play Beatrice. Of sharing books and movies and rants about the news. Of drop-bys and phone calls. Pots of strong coffee. I bet she would have first resisted and then embraced cell phones. And email. She would have loved being able to email photos and updates when she traveled: "That's me on the camel!"

I know it's not unusual to be motherless at fifty-three. I know there are many women who no longer have a mom to borrow clothes from or call for a quick pep talk. But the *if if if* that is so haunting, with Alzheimer's disease, is that there is no one moment when the bells ring out and you realize: This is going to mean saying goodbye. We need to talk about and do and experience everything we've been putting off—now.

Part of the problem is that by the time you know what's going on— *Arlene, we think you have Alzheimer's disease*—it's already too late to do quite a few of those things.

And then one day you look up and realize you've traded places. You're giving the pep talk: "Oh, Mom, don't be silly. We all forget each other's birthdays sometimes—this family is so huge!" You're giving her a sweater because she forgot to bring one. And the stories that never got told? Well, who can think about those now when we have to have conversations about giving up driving or filling the pill-minder or wearing a Safe Return bracelet?

And so the little girls in the photo remain mute. Likewise the pre-teen Arlene holding the trout and the fishing pole. And all the albums full of Mom and Jo Ann, playing and mugging and posing through the years.

Jo Ann and Mom grew apart when they grew up and Mom never really told that story either. It may have had something to do with Jo Ann moving to Texas when she got married and becoming so Texan that she adopted a full-on drawl.

But it's not just Mom and Jo Ann who are mute. There are photo albums in my basement that are more than a hundred years old, full of portraits of veiled brides, stiff-suited grooms, sausage-curled children: some with names—a few that are familiar, many that are not—penciled underneath; many others nameless.

And after Mom moved out of her Madrona house, all of these albums wound up in boxes in my basement.

Where they mutely exist, even when forgotten.

Maybe we Finns are too good at turning our backs on the past. Maybe it was seven centuries of being ruled by Sweden. When Sweden handed Finland over to Russia in 1809 and Russia decreed that Finns would be allowed to speak their own language again, many had to learn it in school. One of those students was a tailor's son and future doctor named Elias Lönnrot, who became so enamored of his new-old language and so concerned about how very little of it existed in writing that he interrupted his medical studies several times to travel the country, collecting and writing down Finnish stories and poems. He began to see patterns, the threads of a Finnish mythology, and he wove the old stories together into an epic poem he called the *Kalevala*, whose dramatic cadence inspired Longfellow's *Hiawatha* and whose fantastic tales, some say, inspired J. R. R. Tolkien's *The Lord of the Rings*.

Lönnrot's name is no longer well known outside of Finland, but he remains a national hero. He gave his people not only a written language but a recorded culture, a unique identity: not Scandinavian, not Baltic, but something different, something ancient, a self-knowledge that the

Finns brought with them when they migrated to the mines and logging camps and fisheries of North America.

One summer Mom finally read Grandma's copy of the English translation of the *Kalevala*, a four-hundred-page tome I now keep on my shelf and have read—some of.

The hero of the *Kalevala* is Väinämöinen, the magic story-singer, who was born an old man, and whose power lay in his amazing memory for every song and story that ever was. He was like the mythic version of Elias Lönnrot: the one who made sure that all the old stories existed, even when forgotten by mere mortals.

Väinamöinen's stories were as powerful as his ability to remember them. He could recite a story and poof! A copper-bottomed boat would appear right when he needed it to get away from some enemy. His stories could make fields flourish or snow melt or the darkness of winter lift from the land. And being hundreds of years old didn't slow him down for a minute.

It's hard not to love a hero like that. Especially if you were an English teacher like Mom and you spent your days trying to persuade teenagers that words are powerful and important.

I wish she'd written down some of her own stories, and some of Grandpa's and Grandma's. But she wasn't blessed with Väinämöinen's centuries or even Elias Lönnrot's eight blazing decades. And all the wishing and What Ifs in the world won't change that.

The other day Nick was loafing around the doorway to my office.

"Mom, what's this?" He picked up a piece of weathered wood from my shelf. "It's been sitting here forever."

"That is not just any piece of wood," I said. I told him that I found it when I went to Red Lodge, Montana thirteen years ago. That I was with Mom and Lisa and we drove around with a map from the county courthouse until we found what we were pretty sure was the farm that Grandma Cere's parents had homesteaded.

"The house was abandoned and we walked around and took pictures and I found that piece of wood outside what looked like it might have been the sauna, which would have been the first thing they built."

"Oh," he said.

"You can see the nail holes in it. Who knows? Maybe my great-grandpa pounded those nails."

That day in Red Lodge, Mom tried so hard to remember the farm. She had visited it many times when she was very young. But it was sold for taxes in 1939, when she was eight years old. Now she was sixty-four and her memories were blowing away like the topsoil of eastern Montana did all through the thirties.

It was on that trip that Lisa and I noticed another strange thing that her brain was doing.

"We saw him yesterday," Mom would declare, pointing to a hitch-hiker on the freeway whom Lisa and I knew none of us had ever seen before in our lives.

"This hotel was great the last time we were here," she would say of a hotel none of us had ever stayed at.

It was as if the sorter mechanism in her brain was misfiring, and new experiences were getting wrongly labeled as memories. As if her brain was trying to compensate for the memories that had gotten trapped in plaques and tangles and were, if not lost altogether, no longer available. As if her brain was working hard to create new stories to fill in for the old ones.

What if someday some scientist as powerful as Väinämöinen figures out how to take that urge that the brain has—to compensate, to do something that works when what used to work no longer does—and uses it to pry loose those trapped memories?

If, if, if it could've happened for Mom.

It didn't.

But what if it could for some other mom? Some other grandma, some other girl with shiny bobbed hair forever frozen in a photo, so much of her story as lost as the Finnish language almost was?

What if?

The Helsinki
Yacht Club

Montana looked beat. Whipped. Ready for a six-month nap under a nice white blanket. It was September 24, 2009 and the edge of that truly big sky that greets you the minute you come out of the Idaho forests was not blue but sooty brown with the smoke of the summer's last stubborn forest fires. The foothill pastures of the Bitterroot Range had gone from golden to silver gray. The cottonwoods along the Clark Fork River wore the faded green of a soldier's oldest pair of fatigues, showing no sign of putting on their fall show. A week from now, a jolt of frost would make them do it. But not yet. Not on this dry, ashy, eighty-degree afternoon.

I was whipped too, after seven solo hours on I-90. Up until the minute I finally got in the car and left Seattle, I had debated whether to make the trip: so many hours of driving; so much to do at home. So wasteful, from a planetary perspective: one person, me, driving from Seattle to Butte, Montana and back: ten hours at least, each way!

So lonesome, the thought of knocking around eerie old Butte by myself.

But I hadn't been there in six years. It was time for an update. If you care about Butte, you need to see it now and then, because bits of it are always disappearing. Which you could say about any place in America, but Butte is a special case.

"In 1955, mining in Butte saw the light, literally," begins the lead story in the Summer 2009 edition of *PitWatch*, a publication of the

Berkeley Pit Public Education Committee. 1955 was the year that the Anaconda Company closed nearly all of its honeycomb of copper mines under Butte and began bulldozing the city's surface. "But," according to *PitWatch*, "mining had always been the lifeblood of Butte, and so the community embraced the new mine, and there was little objection to the sacrifice of some of the city's neighborhoods."

The article goes on to describe how, between 1955 and 1982, the Berkeley Pit, named for one of the shaft mines it replaced, swallowed one neighborhood after another—Meaderville, Dublin Gulch, McQueen, Finntown—until it stretched a mile and a quarter from west to east and a mile from north to south. When mining at the Pit stopped in 1982, the machine-made canyon slowly filled with more than forty billion gallons of contaminated groundwater. Years of environmental litigation ensued. While the lawyers were arguing, scientists found ways to extract the last bits of copper from the wastewater itself.

Now, the Berkeley Pit is part of the biggest EPA Superfund complex of sites in the country—a poison necklace that extends from Butte 120 miles down the Clark Fork River to Missoula. It's a new era in western Montana: if you're drawing a good paycheck, chances are you're an environmental engineer.

Eight hours after I left Seattle, I got off I-90 in Missoula one exit too early. I was distracted by a frightening billboard that featured a photo of a grimy public toilet, with the words: *No one thinks they'll lose their virginity here. Meth will change that.* It was about the tenth Meth billboard I'd seen since the Idaho border.

I found myself in the newest part of Missoula, a neighborhood that had not existed the last time I'd been there, a sprawl of look-alike homes and chain hotels and stores so huge they gave new meaning to the words "big box." Finally I stumbled into the older, more familiar part of town and reached my modest destination, the fifties-vintage Campus Inn, which looked just as beige and worn out as Montana and me.

After I checked in, I went out to stretch my legs. Though I could still smell the forest fires, the evening air revived me. Sandwiched between chain restaurants, I found the River Wok. I took my saffron-steamy

Singapore Noodles back to my room and holed up with a few bottles of Bent Nail IPA from Red Lodge, Montana—purchased in honor of Grandma Cere's birthplace—and Grandma's copy of *Butte's Memory Book*.

Published in 1976, *Butte's Memory Book* is the size of an extra-fat coffee-table book, though it is more like the city's own eccentric photo album than some glossy *PitWatch* kind of publication. It includes a two-page spread on the Pit as it looked in the mid-seventies, when it "had crept to about four blocks from the center of town." But my favorite photos are in the section called "Street Scenes." Most of them are taken in the 1920s, thirties, and forties, when downtown Butte resembled Times Square: every crossing thronged with people, cars, trolleys, but mostly people, all busy, all going somewhere. Eight or ten across on West Park Street at three in the afternoon, according to the clock in one photo from 1941.

Maybe Mom, age ten, is somewhere in that crowd, I thought. Maybe it's a Saturday and Auntie Helen is taking her and Jo Ann out for an ice cream. It looks like a bright, early summer day.

In the foreground of the photo, I spotted a girl with short brown hair walking next to a girl with a mane as glossy and blond as Veronica Lake's. Their backs are to the camera. Their sleeves are puffed and their arms and legs bare. It could be Mom and Jo Ann, who knows? Maybe Auntie Helen couldn't come and they're doing an errand for their grandma, who doesn't like to leave Finntown because she doesn't speak English. They've walked the long blocks from Grandma's house out on the east side and now they're in this crush of people and everyone's got somewhere to go. The Depression's over—Europe is at war—the world needs copper and Butte has the mines and the men for the job.

And, on that fine day in 1941, Butte has children, so many children whose lives are changing even as the photographer snaps his shutter. Their fathers are going back to work.

Their fathers—my grandfather among them—grew up at a time when there was so much good-paying work that it was all a boy could do to stay in school and not bolt for the mines. Grandpa bolted when he was sixteen. Who needed a diploma in 1921 when a strong, healthy teenager could walk away from high school and right down the shaft and be earning what his own father earned in no time at all? In the 1920s, every country in the world needed copper wire, more and more and more of it, to turn the new electric lights on and copper pipes, miles of pipes, to connect all those new faucets and toilets. The Anaconda Copper Company was working three shifts a day to meet the need.

But then, just when Grandpa and his friends were courting and marrying and having their first babies, everything changed.

In 1929, the price of copper plummeted with the stock market and Anaconda started drastically cutting back on production. And a new generation of Butte children, Mom's generation, was born to fathers who worked only some of the time. Fathers who, like my Grandpa, sometimes even took care of the babies and the house while their wives worked as maids. Mom remembered Grandma telling her that Grandpa would pull the shades so no one would see him washing diapers.

That 1941 photo in *Butte's Memory Book* is a picture of a beaten-down city waking up. Even the season is changing: those two girls in the puffed sleeves of summer are surrounded by grownups still in jackets and even coats, still not ready to believe the warm weather's going to last.

I couldn't sleep that night at the Campus Inn. My mind was a jumble of all the photos in *Butte's Memory Book* and all my own Butte memories and all the things I'd left undone at home in order to make the trip. The fan in my room was wheezing like an old miner. I wanted to just turn it off and open my window wide, but I was on the ground floor and all the meth billboards I'd seen on I-90 had made me nervous.

In the morning I went for a shambling run along the stretch of the Clark Fork River that edges the University of Montana's campus. I stopped to read a plaque that proclaimed the riverside trail to be the very route that Lewis and Clark followed two hundred years ago. On this smoky Friday, the most intrepid travelers I passed were a group of barefoot, dreadlocked young people who looked like they'd slept outside.

As I ran, I thought about Mom's one unhappy year as a student here and how the first time I'd visited Missoula I had marveled at the thought of her being unhappy *here* after growing up in Butte: here, on this leafy campus in this velvety river valley, after a childhood on top of a bare hill riddled with belching mines. But Mom had taken a stand against pledging a sorority. She thought sororities were silly and shallow and she didn't realize until it was too late how lonely that would leave her. She began to spend as many weekends as she could at Montana State in Bozeman, four hours away by train, with her high school boyfriend. When John transferred to the University of Washington and her parents announced that they too were moving to a small town near Seattle, Mom followed, thinking she'd resume her studies after a quarter off to earn some money. But it would be twenty years until she went back to school.

The red brick halls Mom knew in 1948 are dwarfed now by a ring of newer, glassier buildings. But the big white, chalk "M" on the side of Mount Sentinel still watches over the campus. And the old bungalows where the professors live are well tended and well gardened and sheltered by the same cozy canopy of oaks and cottonwoods and big-leaf maples that have lined Missoula's streets for a century.

Montanans call Missoula the Garden City, because you can actually grow a garden there: the temperatures are not quite as frigid as the rest of the state and, EPA Superfund complex stretching down the Clark Fork River aside, the dirt in the town itself is not too toxic to grow grass and trees and flowers. But to a girl arriving from Butte in 1948, it might have felt more like a greenhouse than a garden: stuffy, claustrophobic, all dahlias and zinnias and sorority tea parties and country kids from Montana's ranches and farms and forests who hadn't lived through the urban opera of Butte's worst and best years. Kids who thought a crowd meant the county fair, who could not imagine crossing the street in a throng ten deep on an ordinary summer afternoon.

But I wondered, too, as I always do in Missoula: what if Mom had made a few friends and stuck it out at the U of M? She had been such a star student at Butte High School. She had several small scholarships.

And yet, as she wrote in a psychology paper when she finally did go to college two decades later, "My biggest problem lay simply in making decisions . . . By the time I was twenty-one I had married and had my first baby. By the time I was twenty-five I had two babies and a divorce, not of my own choosing. The only goal I can remember having when I was in high school was to complete college, begin a career, and remain single until at least the age of twenty-five. I didn't plan anything; I just let it happen."

I didn't linger in the Garden City. I wanted to get to Butte.

Though I did not set foot in Montana until I was twelve, Butte loomed large over my childhood. We spent a lot of time with our grandparents and one of our favorite things to do was to look at their old photo albums and ask them questions: What is this parade? Who are these people? Grandma, did you really make these Halloween costumes from scratch? As he played solitaire at the kitchen table, Grandpa would throw out cryptic lines about Butte's glory days: about the crowds that greeted visiting presidents and movie stars, mines a mile deep, dance halls that could hold a thousand people, bars full of gambling cowboys and miners.

When I was four, my big sister and brother were picked for a road trip to Butte with Mom, Dad, Grandma, and Grandpa. I was consumed with jealousy: Johnny and Kristie would get to see Butte with their own eyes! Not only that, they would get to sleep at a real motel: the alluringly named Treasure Trails, owned by my grandparents' best friends, Auno and Phil Mikkola.

Finally, when I was twelve and Lisa was ten, it was our turn to go to Butte. But ours would be a different kind of trip: no Dad, because Dad had moved out. Grandpa would drive, with Grandma and Mom next to him in the front seat of Grandpa's cavernous Pontiac and Lisa and I bouncing around in the back, hiding behind the clothes on hangers and taking in, for the first time, the hugeness of the landscape that lay beyond the wet side of the Cascade Mountains.

The Treasure Trails Motel was just as Kristie had described it: like a miniature version of the house on *Bonanza*, with tooled wood and branding irons on the walls and paintings of old Western scenes and a bowl of agates on the front desk and keychains, made from agates, swinging from a little display rack next to the copper bracelets and the postcards. The beds had wool plaid blankets and crisp white sheets. Phil was funny and skinny and Auno was friendly and warm and pillowy. I wanted to stay forever.

This time, all by myself and all grown up, I drove east from Missoula to Butte wishing that the Treasure Trails Motel was still there. But I knew it was long gone, not to the Pit but to the mindless blight of chain hotels and fast-food restaurants that has infected the outskirts of every small city in western America. Phil and Auno were long gone too: like Grandma, like Auntie Helen, like a lot of people in Butte, Auno had died of Parkinson's disease, her big white hands shaking like a cottonwood in a storm.

On this trip, since I couldn't stay at the Treasure Trails, I decided to travel further back in time. I had hoped to stay at the Copper King Mansion, once the home of the mighty copper baron W. A. Clark and now a bed & breakfast inn. I loved imagining what Grandpa or Grandma or Auno or Mom would think if they knew I was sleeping in one of Clark's bedrooms. But I couldn't stay there; the entire mansion was booked by a wedding party. The proprietor suggested I try the Finlen.

Growing up, I had heard stories of the Finlen, which I had always thought was the Hotel Finland, since it was on the edge of Finntown. But no, the nine-story, 1924 landmark was the grandiose project of an Irish businessman named James T. Finlen, who modeled it after the Hotel Astor in New York City. Charles Lindberg, Harry Truman, John F. Kennedy, and Richard Nixon had all stayed there. Historic photos show the bar, the ballroom, the restaurant, the barber shop, the beauty shop, the coffee shop, the grand lobby—all full of people, most of them dressed to the nines.

When I walked in on that Indian summer Friday, it was just the hotel clerk and me, both of us in blue jeans, leaning on the counter under the crystal chandeliers.

She let me look at a few rooms. They were both sixty-eight dollars, twenty bucks less than the Campus Inn back in Missoula. It was hard to choose between the sweeping downhill view to the south, drenched in afternoon sun, or the quieter uphill view of red brick buildings and the gallows frames of the old mines. I chose the uphill view: it would be full of light in the morning and it had an eastern corner window that let in a cooling breeze straight off the Continental Divide.

On Main Street, I found Bob and Sandy's BS Café, sunny and empty, and took a table by the window. The waitress called me "dear." I impulsively ordered a meat and potato pasty, a Butte favorite brought over from Cornwall a century ago by the Cornish miners, who called them "letters from 'ome." My pasty came smothered in gravy, which I hadn't expected and which I knew made it an even worse offender re my little middle-aged cholesterol problem. But the gravy, with its flavor of all the best, crispy bits of roast from the bottom of the pan, reminded me so much of something my grandma would have made forty years ago that it was like a letter from childhood. Like something my tired, solitary self hadn't even known how much it was craving.

After the pasty, I walked, slowly, down the same streets I'd been looking at the night before in the *Butte Memory Book*. It was Friday afternoon. On the busiest blocks, there were maybe half a dozen of us, walking in the sharp shadows of the Metals Bank Building, the M&M Café, the offices and storefronts: many empty, some newly busy with Superfund subcontractors or bead shops or antique stores.

I turned around and headed east on Park Street, crossing Main, towards the blocks where all of my Butte relatives had once lived. Now I was the only person on the street. Now the only business on the block was a thrift shop with a window full of dust-covered baby swings and car seats. Even though a sign said "Open," it was dark and locked.

Then there were no businesses.

Then there were no buildings.

Now I was in the heart of Finntown, which for the last fifty years has resembled the Lower Ninth Ward of New Orleans after Hurricane Katrina: block after block of bare dirt lots with an occasional, lone, broken-down house or a remnant of a foundation. At the end of it all, you arrive at the barbed-wire fences surrounding the Berkeley Pit, where the rest of the neighborhood once was.

There was always one holdout in Finntown: the little white stucco Helsinki Bar, clinging for decades, all alone, to the side of the hill. It was still there, I was happy to see. But as I got closer, I saw that its name had changed since the last time I was in Butte. The new sign said "Helsinki Yacht Club." There were several pickup trucks parked out front. It was, apparently, open.

But I didn't even think of going in. No, I did—it was open and there were people inside—but the sign said "club" and I was a stranger. Though I might feel shy and behave politely, I knew what I would look like, walking in there: a big-city rubbernecker. And who was I to violate the privacy of people who preferred to do their drinking in deep gloom in the middle of the afternoon?

I took a few photos of the exterior. Then I decided to get the car and drive down to the Berkeley Pit viewing stand.

I've been there before, more than once, so it no longer shocks me, this silent canyon that made world headlines in 1995 when 342 migrating snow geese landed on its lethal waters and died within hours. But this time, as I walked through the long white tunnel that leads to the wooden deck overlooking the vast Pit, I felt—something else. Something that I thought might be sadness. My throat was tightening up and I thought I might be about to have a really good cry for my grandparents and my mom and all the other Finns in Butte whose homes and businesses and memories have been chewed up by the Pit. But then I realized that what I felt was not sadness. It was a kind of slow-cooked, well-seasoned anger, an anger that had been simmering on my mental back burner like a strong pan gravy made with toxic wastewater.

Yes, the world needs copper. Yes, I have enjoyed a lifetime supply of electricity and plumbing. But was this really the only way the Anaconda Company could keep the copper coming?

My great-grandfather died at fifty-five of what in Butte was known as the miner's con, short for consumption: coal miners call it black lung. My grandpa died of emphysema. Auntie Helen and Grandma—Parkinson's. Mom—Alzheimer's disease. On the way to Montana, I listened to Mildred Armstrong Kalish's memoir, *Little Heathens*, in which she notes that nearly all of her relatives live healthily into their nineties. Not my family, I thought. Whatever chance we had at that kind of longevity is long buried under that Pit water.

I'm not a scientist, I'm not a doctor, I'm just a writer and a filmmaker who will always wonder why my beautiful, brainy mom wound up with Alzheimer's disease. Staring into the strangely maroon waters of the Berkeley Pit, what took my breath away was not the depth or the circumference of this man-made, poisonous lagoon but the depth and breadth of the greed that dug it, the greed that brought the copper kings and their company heirs to a point where they were willing to first pollute Butte's soil, air, and water beyond recognition and then bulldoze half of it, all for the sake of a profit shared by a very, very few.

I needed a break from sightseeing. I headed back to the hotel.

I thought, as always in Butte, of Hopper and how he would have loved my room at the Finlen at four o'clock on a late September afternoon, with the sun bouncing in off the red buildings across the street. I loved it too; I loved the light and the breeze blowing through. I loved the big dresser and desk and chairs, all dark cherry wood, like something Auntie Helen might have owned.

It occurred to me, as I sipped a strong cup of coffee, that this was the first time I had been to Butte by myself. Maybe that was why the Pit made me so angry this time. I wasn't showing it to my husband or my children, saying, *Can you believe this?* I was seeing it, by myself, without distractions, seeing what it really was.

The first time I stood on that viewing stand was in 1997, on the trip to Montana with Mom and Lisa. We had just come from Red Lodge, where we'd been looking up the homestead farm where Grandma Cere grew up, and now we were in Butte to see what we could find of Mom's roots.

Lisa and I had hoped that being in Butte, or what was left of it, might trigger some childhood memories for Mom. Though we were still a month away from Dr. Forsythe's pronouncement of probable Alzheimer's disease, her memory problems had been getting steadily worse and we felt like if we didn't make the trip that summer, it might really be too late.

But even if your brain is in tip-top shape, it's hard to get much of a trigger out of standing on a weedy lot with nothing to look at but other weedy lots and a big, strangely colored lake that didn't used to be there. Especially if you lived in a dozen different places in your first ten years and nothing is left of a single one of them.

Mom had been to Butte many times during the Berkeley Pit years, so she knew that most of Finntown was gone. But she kept wondering if we were in the right place.

"Well, the Helsinki Bar is still here," she'd say. "So I guess we are. But it just doesn't seem right. Do you think they could've moved the Helsinki Bar?"

A year later, when she returned to Butte with Kristie for her fiftieth high school reunion, she was unable to find her way around the hotel without help.

Five years after that, Rus and I went to her fifty-fifth reunion without her. By that time, she was getting around-the-clock care. Traveling even a few miles in a car was almost impossibly traumatic for her.

Her classmates welcomed us and our camera to the Class of 1948's fifty-fifth Reunion Barbecue at the War Bonnet Motel. They reminisced about how "Arlene was the smartest girl at Butte High School." They asked how she was doing; I told them she was getting really good care and was in good spirits. I didn't tell them that she spoke mostly gibberish and had to be spoon-fed, that her renowned brain now resembled Finntown: a few Helsinki Bar–style holdouts, but overall, not much still standing.

The brick storefronts across the street from my Finlen windows were starting to blaze and shimmer. I went outside to catch the sunset and call home.

I tried to describe to Rus how the old buildings looked like they'd been ignited by the setting sun, how someday he should think of some reason to shoot a film in September in Butte. I told him about the anger I'd felt, staring into the Berkeley Pit after walking the rag-end of Finntown. I thanked him for persuading me to bring a kettle and coffee on this trip: my Finnish forebears would so deeply approve of me brewing up an afternoon cup at the Finlen.

Then I told Rus about the Helsinki Bar and how it was still there but it had changed its name to the Helsinki Yacht Club.

"You have to go in," he said.

I felt that old marital discomfort: bold Rus versus reticent me. But it was a discomfort I well knew was one of the best things about our marriage, though I sometimes pretended otherwise. How many times had he urged me on when I needed urging?

"Are you kidding?" I said. "What if it really is a private club?"

"Well, then they'll tell you it's a private club. But meanwhile, you'll get a look inside."

The sun was resting now on uptown Butte like a fat Cornish pasty on an old iron stove.

"Couldn't I just take a lot of photos of the outside of the bar in this great light?"

Big sigh. "Are you writing a photography book? Go. Just go!"

I told him it looked really grim and depressing, like the kind of place where people drink all day.

"Just go in and order a beer," Rus said. "What's the worst that can happen? It's research. I bet they get people like you all the time, lurking around trying to find their roots."

I watched the sun drop below the horizon and then I walked down the block and into the Helsinki Yacht Club.

It helped that the sun had just set: no more jarring contrast between bright daylight and artificial night, no dismal taint of daytime drinking. But it was dark. Everything was the color of tobacco: the wood of the bar, the barstools, the walls, the air itself, thick with tobacco smoke. Even the dozen or so people inside took on a tobacco hue in the shadowy light, their faces shaded by trucker caps.

The members, if they were members, of the Helsinki Yacht Club ranged from not credibly of drinking age to ancient. Some were standing in groups, some sat or stood at the bar, a few were playing pool. Some looked like they'd just gotten off work and others like they'd been hunched over a shot and a beer all day. I hadn't seen so many people in one place since I got to Butte.

I chose the empty bar stool closest to the open door and ordered a beer, a Montana beer called Moose Drool. Everyone else was drinking Bud or Bud Light and smoking like crazy. Montana was a week away from banning smoking in bars. I wondered if the ban would apply to "clubs."

"Where you from?" asked the bartender as she opened my beer. She was a thirty-something woman with a mane of curly blond hair as thick and healthy as a high school cheerleader's. In fact, she looked like she could once have been a cheerleader—the friendly-wholesome kind, not the bitchy-scary kind.

"Seattle," I said. "But my mom grew up right around here."

"No kidding? You want a glass?"

"No, thanks."

She set the bottle on the bar next to a half-empty bowl of peanuts. "What was your mother's address?"

"Well, they moved a lot. But the address on her birth certificate is 488 ½ East Park Street."

"That's about a block away. We're at 405 East Broadway. My mom will be here soon—she can tell you a lot about the neighborhood."

She plunked four old Polk city directories on the bar. "Have a look."

I opened the oldest one, 1910, and looked up Grundstrom.

And there he was: my great-grandfather, Henry Grundstrom, "top car man, Black Rock Mine, 738 E. Broadway."

Henry Grundstrom. I knew his Omar Sharif eyes and handlebar mustache from one solemn family photo taken when Grandpa was a baby, which would have been five years before this crumbling Polk directory was published. But I never knew he was a "top car man." Did that mean he was in charge of all the car men, whose job was to load the ore into the underground rail cars? Or did that mean he was the best and fastest car man?

I knew, from a copy I had found in Grandma's box of documents, that Henry had "foresworn allegiance to the Czar of Russia" when he became an American citizen, a phrase I loved because it sounded straight out of *Dr. Zhivago*. I knew that he broke his wife's heart when he died in the same year as their daughter. But this little entry in the Polk directory was a snapshot of where he lived and what he did every day. He was a car man, a *top* car man, at the Black Rock Mine. And in 1910, when his youngest child, my grandpa, was five years old, he and Maria and their four children lived at 738 East Broadway.

The cheerleader-bartender leaned over my shoulder and I pointed to his name.

"That's my great-grandfather."

"What's the address? 738? Well, that's definitely in the Pit now."

A short woman with wiry brown hair and a wide, lightly creased face walked in. She wore jeans and an oversized, well-worn, plain blue sweatshirt: an ensemble that said either, "I've been doing housework" or "I really don't care about clothes, never have, never will." I guessed she might be older than me but I really couldn't tell.

"Mom," said the bartender, who looked nothing like her. "Meet Ann from Seattle. She's got roots in the neighborhood. Mom owns this bar," she told me.

"Hi," the short woman said. "I'm Linda. Welcome to the Helsinki Yacht Club. You finding some interesting stuff in there?" Her cell phone rang. "Let me take this call and then I'll show you a great photo that we haven't put on the wall yet."

"Put Frank and Sue on the list," she called out to her daughter, snapping the phone shut. "I'm taking orders for a steak and lobster dinner in a few weeks," she told me. "Twenty-five bucks a couple. How long are you around Butte?"

"Just a few days." The dinner sounded like a great deal. I sincerely wished I could be there. It sounded so casual, so unpretentious, so unlike anything that would ever happen in Seattle.

Linda beckoned me into the smoke and the dark. The pool players paused and up-ended their cues as she led me around the table to the back of the bar and pulled an oversized, black-and-white photo mounted on poster board from behind a partition. Rus was right: no one seemed at all bothered by the sight of a visitor fishing for Finntown roots.

"Let's take it out where we can see it." Linda led me back towards the open door.

We stood outside under the porch light. She held one side of the photo and I held the other. The picture was taken from up the hill, looking down on Finntown and all the other east-side neighborhoods. Block after busy block of apartments, houses, stores—all gone forever.

"There's East Broadway, where we are now. And there's Park. This is where the Pit is now," she added, sweeping her arm across half the picture.

Staring into it, searching for people and laundry and dogs and evidence of lives lived, was a bit like staring at those human outlines I'd seen on the streets of Pompeii and vainly hoping a face will appear, a voice will speak, some miracle will enable us to know what this place was like before all life evaporated. Back when Henry Grundstrom of Raahe, Finland was a top car man who had renounced the Czar. Or when he walked his teenaged son Alton, my grandpa, up to Black Rock to start in the mines. Or when Grandpa, with nothing to do in the midst of the Depression, built his little girls a tiny table and chairs from scrap wood for their pretend-princess tea parties.

"Linda, this is amazing."

It felt like such a pathetic thing to say. Linda didn't seem to mind.

"I know. I know," she said. "Believe it or not, I don't get tired of looking at it."

For a fleeting moment, I felt flooded with envy. As if what I wanted was to *be* Linda, to be living with these photos, these ghosts, in this deserted neighborhood, spending my time fixing up an oddball outpost of a bar where people would flock to my steak dinners.

"I'm curious, are you Finnish?"

She laughed. "Nope, Mexican! But I love this place. I love Butte history. My family goes way back here too. That's what's so great about Butte: what a melting pot it is."

The state of Montana has never been known as a melting pot. But "Butte people," as they call themselves, are not quite Montanan. They're miners, or their parents were, and unlike ranchers and farmers and foresters, miners live close together. People say the old boarding houses used to rent the same bed to two or three miners on different shifts. The miners learned to love each other's food—pasties, tamales, ravioli—and customs: Saturday nights at the Irish saloons followed Saturday afternoons at the Finnish sauna baths. That a short, dark-haired Mexican-American woman with a tall, blonde bartending daughter now runs the Helsinki Yacht Club makes sense in Butte.

"We need to get these things on the walls," Linda said. "I've got some other good photos and then I've got all this nautical stuff. You know, for the yacht club theme."

I still didn't get it.

She smiled. "Because we're on the shores of beautiful Lake Berkeley."

The *PitWatch* newspaper and website does not use the name "Lake Berkeley," although it does call the liquid in the pit "water," as in headlines like, "What's in the Berkeley Pit Water?" or "Montana Resources Mines the Water" or "Research Continues on Pit Water," a fascinating article about unusual Pit-dwelling microbes, known as "extremophiles," that, according to *PitWatch,* may someday be able to prevent migraines or fight cancer.

"In the future, what we can learn from the Pit could represent the greatest treasure of the Richest Hill on Earth," the article concludes.

What we can learn from the Pit. I wonder if that will include anything about Alzheimer's. Or Parkinson's, or the Miner's Con.

The notion of calling the pit Lake Berkeley and calling this little bar the Helsinki Yacht Club—or Bob and Sandy calling their café Bob and Sandy's BS Café—it all fit, somehow, with the sense of humor my mother once had. I could hear one of her favorite pre-Alzheimer's quips about getting older—"I just consider the alternative and then it doesn't bother me"—coming from Linda. Or Sandy, if indeed that was Sandy herself who served me that pasty.

My conversation with Linda kept getting interrupted by regulars who wanted to get on her list for the steak and lobster feed and other regulars who had comments on the state of the pool cues or the jukebox and others who just wanted to say hi. During the interruptions, I found more Grundstrom listings in the 1916 (Henry, Maria, and family, 540 East Broadway) and 1948 (Alton, Cere, and family, 1826 Adams, down on the Flats at last in their own little house) directories.

Tiny, tiny bits of type on a thin page. Nothing, nothing at all compared to a photo or one of Grandpa's scraps of super-8 film. Nothing compared to a remembered scrap of story from Mom or Grandpa or Grandma. And yet I felt almost seasick, as if I had a new pair of glasses on that were much stronger than the old pair and I could suddenly see: in those cryptic Polk listings I could see the streets, the homes, where my mother's life had started. Where her father's life had started. Where old Henry Grundstrom, who never actually was old, began something: a new-world family.

"The cradle rocks above an abyss, and common sense tells us that our existence is but a brief crack of light between two eternities of darkness," Vladimir Nabokov writes, in the opening words of his memoir, *Speak, Memory*. Sitting on my stool at the bar of the Helsinki Yacht Club, I felt like I had been given a flashlight that, just for a moment, could see backwards into the darkness.

But of course I couldn't say any of this, not to these Butte people who were so used to living in a ghost town. A ghost city. A ghost melting pot.

I behaved like a good Finn and stayed quiet.

In the 1957 directory (long after my grandparents had left for Buckley, Washington), I found the Treasure Trails Motel. I showed the address to Linda.

"Do you know what's there now?" I asked.

She closed her eyes for a minute. "Let's see, 3440 Harrison: that would be down on the Flats, across from the Hampton Inn—you know what?" She smiled.

"What?"

"I think it's a casino called the Treasure Chest. I wonder if they named it that on purpose."

151

The next morning, I drove down Harrison looking for the Hampton Inn and the Treasure Chest.

When I finally spotted it, I felt some of that slow-burning anger I'd felt at the Pit viewing stand. It was such an ugly little building. It didn't even look like a casino, let alone a casino deserving of the name *Treasure Chest*. It looked like an insurance office or a cut-rate dental clinic or maybe a place you'd go to buy something you wished you didn't have to buy, like a wheelchair or an oxygen tank.

I was in Billings once for work and I found a place to stay that reminded me of the Treasure Trails. It was called the Dude Rancher and it had the same *Bonanza* décor and the same cozy feel. I remember that it started to snow, tiny dry flakes swirling outside my room and rapidly coating the knotty pine windowsill. It was early October. It reminded me of that old story Mom liked to tell about a million times too often about the day it snowed in June and the Butte kids got to stay home from school. Maybe it got stuck in her mind because she liked the theme, which seemed to be that Butte was the kind of place where crazy things happened, like snow days in June.

Or a yacht club on the shores of Lake Berkeley.

That Park Street address on my mother's birth certificate, just downhill from the Helsinki Yacht Club—488 ½ East Park—that was where Grandpa lived with his mother and brother Niilo in 1930, according to the federal census from that year. They paid twenty dollars in rent to the owners, Auntie Helen and her husband Albert, who lived in the apartment next door. My great-grandpa Henry had died in 1926. Grandpa's sister Jemina died within months of their father's death, of influenza or some other sudden killing illness of the era. I don't remember and there's no one left for me to ask. So in 1930, the Grundstrom family consisted of Grandpa, his heartbroken mother, his brother, who was in poor health and died a short time later, and Auntie Helen and her husband. Grandpa and Grandma hadn't married yet.

My mom was born on March 25, 1931. 488 ½ E. Park was her first address.

I wish I knew something about her birth. I wish Grandma had told me a story that started, "The day your mother was born . . . "

The day your mother was born, it snowed tiny flakes like stars that could fit on the head of a pin.

I love all the pictures Grandpa took of Mom as a baby, looking so chubby and jolly that you'd never guess there was a Depression going on.

Your mom's big baby smile lit up the house. She made Grandpa's mother smile for the first time in five years.

I love the way Grandma looks in those pictures too: her smile just as big and joyous as baby Arlene's. Her youth so surprising.

The summer your mother was a baby, we took her to the farm in Red Lodge to meet my family. Nothing soothed her like the roar of Rock Creek. We picnicked by the boiling rapids every day. I thought we'd all be deaf in two weeks! Grandpa fished for trout. We ate as much as we wanted and your mother grew as fat as a little cupid.

But Grandma never talked like that.

Like Mom, she'd been a standout scholar, earning the highest score in her county on the eighth grade graduation exam. But when she was thirty-five, she almost died of encephalitis, and she never again felt the mental sharpness on which she'd prided herself as a young woman. In her final years, Parkinson's shot its shaky tendrils through her brain. She often thought she was back on the farm in Red Lodge and called me by one of her four sisters' names when I came to visit.

I wondered so often where Mom was in her final years. I often thought of Grandma and wished that Mom, too, could mentally transport herself to a grassy homestead farm just downriver from Yellowstone.

I feared that Mom was somewhere scarier. That she was caught in a cold white passageway, like the tunnel to the Berkeley Pit viewing stand.

Maybe not. Maybe she was laughing and sledding on a snow day in June.

Or maybe she went back to her baby self. Maybe her brain played the loud symphony of the Rock Creek rapids, lulling her to a deep and deafened sleep, allowing her to rest at last after all those years of struggling to stay afloat on a rising lake of toxic plaques and tangles.

153

Maybe she found her own Helsinki Yacht Club. Her own dark, cozy respite from the wasteland of her shrinking brain. Where her grandpa, whom she never knew, wasn't dead of the miner's con, he was a strapping, strong Finn who had risen to be the top car man at the Black Rock Mine. Where she and her mother were both still young women, still smiling, still sharp as two brass tacks. I could just see them hanging Linda's photos of Finntown on the walls of the Yacht Club and debating where to put the nautical stuff: the buoys and ropes and life rings that would never be needed to fish anyone out of Lake Berkeley, where no one who had a brain would ever swim.

Driving away from Butte the next day, I decided to stop at Gregson, as my Grandma used to call it. In her day, Gregson was a place where the steam-loving Finns and all the other tired miners could soak away the afternoon in the waters of the natural hot springs. Now, the springs have been tamed into a series of pools called the Fairmont Hot Springs Resort.

I paid my eight dollars and slipped into the ninety-four-degree "lap pool," where I swam slowly, back and forth, stretching, switching strokes, letting the anger and sadness and lostness of Butte slip away for at least this little while. Then I switched to the 101-degree soaking pool, resting my head on the edge, basking in the last minutes of Montana's summer, thinking of nothing. When I got too warm, I would get out for a minute and sit in the cool fall breeze that had kicked up overnight and watch the tumbleweeds blow through the meadow outside the Fairmont's fence. Then I'd slip back in for just a few more minutes.

I had only driven fifteen of the five hundred miles home.

Northern House

Trying to find a home for someone who's done a stint at the Seattle Geropsychiatric Center is like trying to find a home for a paroled sex offender. We weren't yet accustomed to thinking of our mother as a parolee, an ex-con of the dementia world. So we were grateful for Northern House.

We knew how hard Lynette, the Gero Psych social worker, had labored to find this new address for Mom after it became clear that she would no longer "fit in" at Fairview Terrace. But that didn't mean we didn't notice things, like the split-level, floor-plan-in-a-can dreariness of the place; the peeling, Kleenex-blue paint; the faint lines of moss creeping up the outside walls; the cloying floral furniture you wouldn't wish on your most impoverished college-aged nephew.

Mom loved good woods, strong stripes, straight lines. She would never have chosen Northern House in a million years.

And yet, it was surrounded by tall trees, some of them probably 150 years old: big, patient, second-growth Douglas firs miraculously left standing when the split-level people came through forty or fifty years ago. And it was tucked into a winding ravine in a neighborhood just north of the Seattle city limits, not too far from the little red ranch house that she and Dad bought when they were newlyweds. Sometimes I took the old highway to get there instead of the freeway and drove past landmarks Mom would have loved: Highland Ice Arena, where she, who had grown up skating in Butte, held out her hands and coaxed us away from the edge of the rink; Leilani Lanes, where she dropped off me and baby Lisa in the upstairs nursery and I watched her through the big glass

155

window, looking so serious as she stared at those pins and then twirling into her huge, happy smile after the crash of a strike, which I still think is one of the best noises in the world.

The round-the-clock staff at Northern House radiated calm and kindness and tree-like patience. Most of them were from Gambia or Ethiopia, and you got the feeling that taking care of people with brain damage and dementia was a breeze compared to some of the earlier chapters of their lives.

They had a completely new view of Mom: the view of people who had never known her any other way.

Before Seattle Gero Psych, in her two years at the Lakeview Retirement Community, she had gone from hosting illicit wine parties and modeling at the annual fashion show to yelling at the staff when they tried to call her out of her room for meals and flat-out refusing to bathe. But the caregivers at Northern House had not seen any of that transformation. Nor had they seen her tied to a wheelchair in the Gero Psych dayroom. They only knew her as the gnomish white-haired woman who walked up and down the hallway all day, muttering and gesturing, but never tiring herself enough to sleep; who looked closer to ninety than she did to her real age, seventy; who had four blue-eyed daughters who were impossibly hard to keep straight. They didn't wince at having to cut up her food and feed her with a spoon because they didn't know that just a few months ago, she'd been feeding herself just fine. They didn't mind if she yelled through her shower because they knew she'd be calm afterwards, soothed by the warm towel and the brush running through her bobbed hair. Arlene didn't have the thatchy old-lady hair of the other women at Northern House; hers was as fine and straight as her many daughters'.

Unlike the Lakeview or Seattle Gero Psych, Northern House was a last-stop destination. No one pretended that anyone there would ever be well enough to live anywhere else, not even the two youngish residents. One was a brain-damaged car accident victim who was under thirty. The other was in his forties and had inherited Creutzfeldt-Jakob disease (known in its infectious form as Mad Cow disease), which, his wife said, was rapidly turning his brain into Swiss cheese. Then there was Jon, who was nearing 100, had no family left, and spoke to everyone in Norwegian because, after eighty years in America, he could no longer remember a word of English. And then there were the two downstairs ladies: one didn't speak or eat and was fed through a stomach tube and the other was a skeletal wisp who was quietly weepy most of the time but every now and then would let out a series of screams that rocked the house.

And then there was Mom.

Through the looking glass of her disastrous five days at Fairview Terrace followed by the zombifying dose of Haldol and the slow detox at Seattle Gero Psych, Mom had slipped into the late stage of Alzheimer's. Outings were now too exhausting and overwhelming. My sisters and I no longer got to play the role of liberators, signing her out, as we had at the Lakeview, for family birthday parties or walks or restaurant meals. Now we were visitors. We brought chocolate and photos and flowers from our gardens. We emailed each other constantly, comparing notes about when we planned to visit so that Mom would have visitors on as many different days as possible, then sending updates about how she was doing when we saw her.

"Anyway, re: my Mom visit last Sat., she seemed OK, much the same. She was very talkative, almost nonstop with a mix of pure gibberish, words that made no sense, and little snippets of meaningful conversation . . . "

"So like a baby now it amazes me. She enjoys eating so much . . . "

I often came at lunchtime because feeding her gave me something to do. Sometimes she was happy to see me. Other times, she didn't seem to know me. Sometimes she liked it when I sat next to her on the couch and put my arm around her as if I was a teenage boy and she was my girlfriend. Sometimes she liked it when I sang songs, the oldest songs I could think of, songs I remembered her father singing, like *Darling Clementine.* Whether she was treating me like a daughter or a stranger on any particular day did not seem to have anything to do with how well she liked my cuddling or my laughable singing or the food I was feeding her.

She grew tired and cranky if I stayed too long. At least that's what I told myself, as I watched the clock tick while I sang, talked, spooned macaroni, all the while feeling like some kind of desperate performance artist who just couldn't get the audience to wake up and was now counting the minutes until I could run from the stage. *Herring boxes without topses, sandals were, for Clementine . . .*

Maybe my sisters and I shouldn't have been so strict about not visiting on the same days. But we knew that if we were there at the same time, we would be tempted to just talk to each other and ignore Mom and also that it would mean she might not get a visitor on another day. Northern House was not a quick drive for any of us: twenty-five or thirty minutes each way for me or Caroline, an hour and a half each way for Lisa or Kristie.

And, we reasoned, it was good for Mom in a general sense if the staff knew that one of us might stroll in any old time.

What we didn't know is how much any of it mattered to Mom.

There are so many kinds of loneliness. There's the eerie isolation of being packed into a subway or walking down a crowded street where no one dares to make eye contact. Or the pressing in of the walls when you're alone in a new town and have no one to call. But I've never felt as lonely in all my life as I did when I visited my mother at Northern House. To sit across the table from the person who was the very first person I loved, the very first person to love me; to try with all my might to will her eyes to meet mine and then to have to give up, to accept her eyes not seeing me—and then to have one of her well-meaning caregivers comment on how pretty Arlene looks today, her lovely skin, her clean white hair—I wanted to shout, Who cares? She's gone! Can't you see that this is not Arlene, this is an old-woman rag doll who we are all pretending is still a living person? Can't you see that the reason I have to leave the very minute the clock strikes the hour is not that I have so much work to do, which is what I always say, but because I have to get in my car and drive down the street until I'm out of your sight and then I can stop and let out this sob I've been strangling on for the last half hour?

This went on for four years.

At each visit, there was another downhill step, another bit of bad news to report: She won't chew her food. We have to put her in a diaper. She won't stand up straight. She won't stand up at all. Four years: from walking and muttering to limp and mute in a wheelchair, all connections between brain and muscles severed.

Lost and gone forever, dreadful sorry, Clementine.

And during those four years, the visits to Mom were sandwiched between all the rest of my life, just as they were for my sisters and for my brother when he visited from New Jersey. "Sandwiched": it sounds so easy, a simple matter of tucking the ham in between the bread and the lettuce. But it never was. It was never easy to tuck a known mood-wrecker into the day; to know that I was going to get up from my desk, get in my car and drive into a wall, again, and then recover, again, like the world's most resilient crash test dummy. It was never easy to do it, not knowing how many months or years I was going to keep doing it, which meant I couldn't have a big breakdown every time, I just couldn't; it wouldn't be fair to my husband or children or friends or workmates.

So I learned what I needed to do to smother the sadness and get on with the day. I stopped for the sob down the block from Northern House, and then, if I had time, I did some transitional something between the visit with Mom and having to function in the world of my daily life. Sometimes, I went to Third Place Books, over the hill from Northern House. If I felt too wrecked to browse books, I would browse magazines in their café over a bowl of soup, a practice the store graciously allowed. If I felt like I should do something that could be construed as useful, I stopped at Trader Joe's or Costco and loaded up on groceries. There were a few friends I could walk with or have lunch with immediately after visiting Mom and I could either talk about her or not.

But there were many people I felt I could not see or talk to right after seeing her. My dad and stepmom, for example. They couldn't help being healthy and athletic and youthful; it was irrational of me to think of their good fortune as somehow "unfair." But here they were, flying back and forth to Phoenix for their tennis and golf and sunshine while Mom lived out her shredded life at Northern House. And here I was, that old divorce scar tissue flaming up whenever Dad asked, "How's Arlene?" I knew it made no sense. And yet it was true.

Maybe all grave illnesses do this to families: bring up old hurts, inflame old wounds. But Alzheimer's disease has its own particularly insidious torture methods. One is the open-endedness of it. There is no three month, six month, couple-of-years-if-you're-lucky kind of diagnosis like you might get with cancer. It could be a year or a decade. Or two decades. Mom's body was strong. So I couldn't afford not to tamp down the sadness after my visits. I couldn't allow myself to lash out at Dad for no currently relevant reason. I couldn't ask for sympathy or breaks from colleagues or clients or friends, because what if I found myself needing even more sympathy or bigger breaks down the road?

I had to conserve emotional energy.

Another of Alzheimer's tortures is that once you've passed a certain point, you can no longer talk about it with the person who has it. There is no crying together about the awfulness of fate; there are no good-byes. If Mom was raging against her illness somewhere deep inside, we didn't know it. She couldn't tell us.

I wondered often, at Northern House, if she was. Raging. If her pacing and muttering and later, in the wheelchair, her sudden bursts of incoherent agitation were her ways of trying to say, Why? Why can't you get me out of here, out of this prison? Why can't someone or something or some drug get in here and clear a path through my brain?

She couldn't tell us whether she was tired or not, but she always looked exhausted. Whipped, like Montana at the end of a parched summer. Like just existing in a world she could no longer make sense of was harder than anything she had ever done. Alzheimer's disease, or at least my mom's Alzheimer's disease, is not some peaceful, slow fade-out; it's a futile struggle against quicksand, an instant of suffocating panic stretched out over years and years and years.

But it's not like I could go around talking about this, especially when Mom was still alive. No one wants to hear these kinds of things about an illness that afflicts five million Americans and twenty-six million people worldwide. No one wants to imagine that much suffocating panic going on all over our planet.

So, especially right after seeing Mom, I tried to avoid people who were likely to ask well-meaning questions like, "How's your mom doing?" I tried to stay very far away from the people who I knew would give me that look that said, "I'm asking how your mom is doing but I am hoping your answer will be really short because I'd rather talk about rabies or herpes or toxic slime than Alzheimer's disease," or the people who I felt had already judged me for having put her in a "home" instead of caring for her in my own home, or the people who said things like, "Well, I certainly have my share of Alzheimer's moments—you should have seen me looking for my keys this morning!"

Sometimes after seeing Mom I had to just drive straight home and have a good cry on Rus's shoulder. But I tried not to do it too often because I didn't want him to worry that I was falling apart—especially considering that this might go on for years—and I also didn't want to blow up his day.

Rus and I had talked a few times about making a documentary film about Mom. My sisters were wary. I was wary. We tried shooting a little bit once, on her sixty-eighth birthday, in 1999. But when Rus asked, "Arlene, how old are you today?" and then filmed her trying to laugh off the fact that she had no idea—I felt—well, I felt something like what I felt when he and I took a day job with a tabloid TV show and staked out Kurt Cobain's house after Cobain shot himself. I was ashamed. I wanted to shower. I called my sisters the next day and told them not to worry, we weren't going to make a film about Mom.

But the world was different in 2002. Mom was at Northern House, her ability to laugh at herself or anything lost and gone forever. And George Bush was president.

When Bush announced his decision to restrict stem-cell research to a uselessly small pool of available stem cell lines, and then Laura Bush sanctimoniously opined that even though her father had Alzheimer's disease, she was 100 percent behind her husband's decision, some little switch flipped inside me. I wrote a guest editorial and sent it to the *Seattle Post-Intelligencer*.

"Much is Lost to Alzheimer's Disease" was the headline that the P-I put on it. "I see my Mom often, yet every time I see her, I miss her even more," I wrote. "She is moving into the late stage of Alzheimer's disease, a slow killer that has robbed me, my brothers and sisters, our children, and all the other people whose lives my mother's life touched of the beautiful, intelligent woman we knew . . . You might say, 'Get over it. It's sad, but there are worse things. Seventy-one is hardly young.' Perhaps that's what President Bush would say to me, as he explains why he can't support the stem-cell research that could be crucial to our understanding of Alzheimer's and other brain diseases."

Friends and family and total strangers responded warmly. It felt good. It felt like a way to un-smother the sadness without hurting anyone and, who knows, maybe even helping somehow: not Mom, but other people like me and my siblings who were logging their own lonely hours visiting someone they loved who no longer knew who they were. Or all the people who were caring fulltime for someone with Alzheimer's disease. Or all the scientists working long hours in a research lab, with or without stem cells.

I began to think again about the idea of making a documentary. Rus and I had been making more and more short films together, mostly for non-profits, and we had some new ideas about how we could go about it. We agreed that it would not be a visual chronicle of Mom's downhill slide, that we would shoot very little footage of Mom with Alzheimer's. Instead, we would use photos and old home movies and videos. We would make it personal but also journalistic; we would find scientists and doctors to interview. We would shoot it over one year, 2003, fitting it in with our other work. Because we owned all our own gear, we could do it without having to raise production money. We would just do everything ourselves. It would be a good change from working for clients; it would be good to write in my own voice. It would be a way to channel the sadness. To use it.

I called the University of Washington's Alzheimer's Disease Research

Center, full of questions, hoping to line up some interviews. The administrator surprised me with a question of her own.

"Why don't you volunteer for research?" she said. "As a control subject. It could be part of your film."

And so I found myself in a room at Seattle's huge VA Hospital, where the Alzheimer's Disease Research Center is located, taking all the memory tests I'd watched Mom flunk. The tests start with questions like, *What day is it? Who is the president?* and progress through tasks like spelling "world" backwards, listening to a paragraph and recalling details ten minutes later, repeating back sequences of numbers, remembering short lists of words, distinguishing the words for colors from the actual colors, going back to that paragraph and recalling it again, going back to those numbers and doing the sequences in reverse order. There were neurological tests too, in which I was tickled with feathers, tapped on the elbows and knees, peered at with a penlight in my eyes. And there were psychological questions: *On a scale of one to ten, do you usually feel life is worth living?*

I was weighed and measured. I gave blood. I peed in a cup. My family tree was drawn, with special attention to anything that might be relevant: Grandma Cere's Parkinson's disease; Great Aunt Eine's Alzheimer's disease, which started in her seventies. I was approved for a lumbar puncture, more commonly known as a spinal tap, and a week later, I came back and curled up in a ball while two tablespoons of fluid were extracted from my spine with a long quivery needle: two tablespoons that would be turned into fifty droplet-sized samples for research. Rus filmed nearly all of it, from *What day is it?* right through the spinal tap. Later, we filmed interviews with four different doctors. Later still, we interviewed my sisters and our daughter.

It didn't make visiting Mom any easier. Most days, I still left with a sob stuck in my throat. But I was doing *something* and that was so much better than *nothing*, the big helpless Nothing I brought to Mom when I visited her, lost in her cavern in a canyon; Nothing served up with maybe a little pudding on a spoon and another verse of *Clementine*.

Because we had to fit the work on the documentary into our work that paid the bills, we didn't finish it until spring of 2004. And all through those many months, Mom continued to ebb away.

I can't remember exactly when she stopped walking; I do remember that it seemed sudden. That she went almost overnight from logging a dozen miles a day, up and down the hallway, to never moving again. That once her legs refused to walk, that was it, as if the walking center in her brain had just been sealed off. Like the vision center: she no longer seemed able to see anything flat—a photo, a painting in an art book. Or the language center: the words that spilled out of her now were bits of confetti, tiny scraps, as if the sealed-off language center had maybe one tiny opening, one mousehole-sized door—but alas, it also contained a shredder.

Mom's brain was being walled in brick-by-brick towards death, like Fortunato in Poe's story, *The Cask of the Amontillado*: an allusion she, the English teacher, would have liked much better than poor old Clementine.

In the earlier stages of Alzheimer's disease, I didn't think of her as dying. We all are, I know, whether we wear the label of an illness or not. But the fashion now is to say *living with*, not *dying of*, as in, "He is living with cancer," or diabetes, or heart disease. When Mom was first diagnosed, it wasn't hard to think of her as *living with* this condition called Alzheimer's disease: though her memory was impaired, she was still very lively and alive. Even when she first moved into Northern House, pacing and grumbling, I did not think of her as dying. Not the way she walked the halls and polished off her meals. But as 2002 became 2003, 2004, 2005, as walking and talking and seeing all got bricked off and Mom seemed to be visibly shrinking, slumping ever further into her wheelchair, even her spine going slack—I began to feel this other presence in the room. Death. Parked quietly on the couch like a polite guest who is content to wait his turn to speak. No hurry. Please, go on.

In the documentary film *Stranded: I've Come from a Plane That Crashed on the Mountains*, the sixteen survivors of the infamous 1972 plane crash high in the Andes speak eloquently about what it was like to live in close quarters with death for ten weeks. About how preferable death seemed, at the time, to being alive and stranded in an Andean valley full of nothing but snow. The infamy of their story comes from what they did to survive: they ate the frozen bodies of their friends. But in the interviews filmed thirty years later, they don't use the word the rest of the world used, *cannibalism*, to describe what they did. They use words like *communion. Sharing. What we had to do.* They talk about portions laid out and consumed in silence. They never call what they ate meat or flesh; they call it food. They talk about how, when they look at the children they have raised because God allowed them to live, they feel their dead friends with them.

They speak vividly about viewing the other side of death when an avalanche buried the plane two weeks after the crash and they all thought they were dying. How beautiful it was. How they longed to go there. How hard it was when their mouths found air and they realized their destiny was not to die yet.

I watched *Stranded* a few nights ago and I wondered again what I always wonder when I think about Mom dying: did she get to see the light, the beauty?

And as I listened to the stories of the sacred food, consumed solemnly with only one purpose—life—I thought of Mom's last weeks. How all that was left for her was the swallowing of food: the powerful human urge to stay alive, past all sensible end points, all logic.

It seemed she could still taste. Chocolate, always chocolate, would make her seek the spoon like a blind bird. She, who had fed so many babies, who for fifty years had urged children and grandchildren to eat and grow, now sought her own last spoonfuls of nourishment, her own last portions of life.

Some people, nearing death, stop eating. Not Arlene.

Not until a cold turned into pneumonia and she had to focus on trying to breathe.

It was the first weekend of March, 2006. I was in Sarasota, Florida, showing our film, *Quick Brown Fox: An Alzheimer's Story*—her film—at the United Nations Women's Film Festival, called "Through Women's Eyes." I didn't know yet about Mom's cold, but I was so stuffed up I could barely breathe myself. I loaded up on decongestant for the screening and Q&A. This was not the first time I had shown the film but it felt new and so right to be in a women's festival. It was something Mom would have loved: all these creative, dynamic women together in a bright, coastal place, sharing their films and stories. *Quick Brown Fox* was received very warmly.

But for two nights, I couldn't sleep at all in Florida. I was staying in the lovely, bougainvillea-draped, stucco home of one of the festival organizers, and she was so kind and attentive and worried about my miserable cold; how could I tell her that I was also having the worst insomnia of my life? Puny scraps of sleep, scraps of dreams. Mom was in my dreams but that was not remarkable because she always was. Besides, all weekend long I'd been talking about *Quick Brown Fox*, which meant I'd been talking and thinking about her.

At last I was driving across that long bridge over Tampa Bay towards the airport and home. I had just left the sunshine and turned into the climbing tunnel of the rental car garage when my phone rang. It was my sister Lisa, calling to tell me that Mom had pneumonia and when would I be home?

I drove up to Northern House that night. My brother James and youngest sister, Caroline, were there. Kristie and Lisa had gone home but would be back the next day. Mom was in bed, lying on her side, breathing like an old mountain train. She had an oxygen pump and morphine. Her eyes were closed but she was perspiring, focused, in a state other than sleep.

"You guys go," I said. "I'll stay a while."

Caroline and James urged me not to feel like I had to stay all night. The hospice nurse had said it could be several more days.

I put some couch cushions down next to Mom's bed and lay down. I was so tired. I stroked her hand and talked to her; I babbled a little about the festival. I drifted in and out of sleep.

Sometime in the wee hours of the morning, I woke up. Mom was still breathing noisily but she seemed to be asleep.

The overnight caregiver peeked in.

"It will be many days," he said. "I know how strong your mother is. And I have seen this many times."

I was crying. "I'm sorry. I'm crying because I'm so exhausted."

"Go home," he said. "Go rest."

I nodded and wiped my eyes. Yes, I thought. He is right. I'm being ridiculous. This could be a long haul and I need rest.

I got up and drove home and collapsed into bed next to Rus for about two hours.

The ringing phone woke us at six. It was Kristie. She was calling from Northern House. Mom was dead.

Mom was dead. I had left her in her final few hours. Mom had died alone.

I can barely stand to write those words. I can barely stand the thought of my mother having to die alone because I stumbled out of her room at three something in the morning and drove home to my bed and my husband and my life while she breathed her last breaths alone. She worked so hard to stay alive as long as she did and her reward was to die alone. She had six children and fourteen grandchildren and she died alone.

Some hours later, I called my minister and friend, Lee, from Northern House, to tell him Mom had died. And that she had died alone. Because I left.

"I've seen this so many times," Lee said. "The family gathers, people fly in from far away, like you did and James did, and then the minute everyone leaves the room, the dying person is able to let go. It's almost like they've been waiting to be alone. Like death is a passage that many of us need to make alone."

I don't know if this is true, or if Lee just knew I needed to hear something that would help me. But it did help; it helped so much. I won't ever quite forgive myself for leaving that night but if Lee's right, maybe Mom forgave me long ago. Maybe after all those years in the prison of Alzheimer's disease, her soul longed to stand alone and step off the edge of the world, free of anything that might tempt her to stay another second—and that might have been my breath, my touch, still pulling on her ever so gently, just when she was ready to fly off into the light.

Because wouldn't she see it, after all? Letting go of her body, her physical wreck of a brain, wouldn't her soul get to see all that light?

I hope it was as warm as the light in Florida. As clear and pure as the Rocky Mountain camping trips of her childhood. As dazzling as the pink evening glow on Mt. Rainier over Lake Washington, which was her favorite view in all of this world, though it might be nothing much compared to what those who have come close say they've seen waiting for us on the other side.

Whatever it is, I just want her to see it and feel it and be it. Be light, nothing but light, after all those years in the dark.

Epilogue: Light She Was

"Light she was and like a feather
And her shoes were number nine;
Herring boxes without topses,
Sandals were for Clementine."

L ike a feather: that's how I remember singing the song, though I think the real words were "like a fairy," which is funnier, especially considering that her shoes were size nine.

Light she was and like a feather. And now, whatever her faults—big feet, funny sandals—Clementine is lost. Gone forever. That's what the song mourns: that she was light and that she is now lost.

There are some people who are going to read this book and say, There are a lot of things you left out.

For example: I left out how Mom didn't take me to the doctor for three days after I broke my wrist when I was seven because she thought I was exaggerating.

I left out how she would put down my dad in front of the other guests at a party if she knew something about literature or history that he didn't.

I left out how blinded she was by my older brother's brilliance. How she was so focused on John, the math genius, that she didn't always see John, the angry little boy.

169

I left out how her liberal politics did not match her love of the Tennis Club lifestyle.

I left out the colossal sobbing fight she and I had one night in the middle of Second Avenue in downtown Seattle after a meal, paid for by her, in which I accused her of taking no interest in my life. It was 1986. I had recently left my husband and I was dating this new guy, Rus, and she seemed utterly uncaring, or so I thought at the time.

Now I look back and think, Was she already struggling just to stay on top of the wave of information she had to remember every day? 150 high school students' names? The new principal's latest new rules?

And why wouldn't I leave all of that out? Why wouldn't I prefer to dwell on how light she was?

How light she was. How her smile could lift me, feather light, right out of the caverns of adolescent gloom.

How lightly she wore the busyness of her life: never complaining, just moving through her day like the world's calmest air traffic controller, constantly sweeping the sky, readying the next plane to launch or land. We all grew up aware that we were each just one of six little planes on her screen. But we also grew up knowing that she would never forget us, never let us drop off the radar and crash. Without dwelling on it, we relied completely on her talent for zeroing in on our needs at any given moment.

In that paper she wrote for a psychology class that she took not long after she went back to school in the middle of her life, Mom laughed off the notion of mothering as a "skill." "For me, it's easy to have children and to love them, and no great thought or effort goes into rearing them. I just do what I have to do," she wrote forty years ago. "When people mention my abilities as a mother, I feel fraudulent." (No one said "parenting" back then; I'm not sure anyone even said "mothering" very often.) She insisted that whatever parental talent she possessed was completely instinctual—"no great thought or effort"—but lucky for us, her instincts were remarkably good.

She snapped to attention, for example, when I came home at the end of my freshman year of college, encased in about thirty extra pounds, and told her I thought maybe I needed to see a counselor because I was having moments where I didn't quite see the point of living. She sent me to a psychiatrist named Dr. Ottosen, a funny name that I will love forever. He was in a fancy office tower and wore perfectly tailored blazers and I'm sure he was expensive but Mom told me not to worry.

Dr. Ottosen listened and listened and then he said the simplest things that somehow helped me change the way my brain worked. He taught me that I could accept and even embrace contradictions rather than letting them eat me up. He taught me that I not only deserved to, but also *needed* to, love myself whether or not any boy currently did. What this meant in practice was that I could go ahead and love my dad even though he'd done some things I hated, and I could love my brother even though he had been such a terrible bully, and I could love myself even though I'd gained a couple of sleeping bags' worth of weight. Maybe I would have figured all of that out eventually. But Mom saw my neediness and she saw that I might crash, and I was forever grateful to her for taking me seriously.

She took me seriously again when Claire was born and my feelings of isolation and panic caught me by surprise. Effortless though she claimed motherhood to be, she apparently had not forgotten her own first months, when maybe she wasn't yet so ultra-sure of her instincts. Maybe she too had felt isolated with a new baby in a small apartment, her husband and neighbors and friends gone all day.

She knew that what I needed was company, mainly: patient company, someone to make me laugh while I struggled with the car seat and the overly collapsible stroller and the diapers and the endless, endless feeding. She knew I needed someone to appreciate Claire's quirks and incremental changes. The babies born in our extended family in the couple of years right before Claire were angelic and quiet, so Claire got labeled "fussy" by everyone but Mom, who often was able to magically soothe her and when she couldn't, was happy to bounce, rock and roll along with her baby moods.

There is one day I love to remember as much as I love the name "Ottosen." It was a silly day, inconsequential; who knew that I would love the memory of it the way I do? A warm July day, Claire was still just a handful of weeks old, and Rus was working. Mom and I decided to go to the Northgate Mall: the mall of my childhood, an old and unpretentious mall in north Seattle anchored, as it still is, by a Nordstrom store at one end and a Penney's at the other. She drove across town from her Madrona house to my apartment on Queen Anne Hill. We struggled together down the three flights of stairs with Claire, the car seat, the stroller, the diaper bag. We worked together to figure out the best way to fit it all into Mom's little Tercel, which seemed like a better bet than my VW bug.

By the time we got to Northgate, all three of us were starving.

"Let's go to the restaurant in Penney's," Mom said. "They've got booths. You can nurse there."

"Mom, I haven't nursed yet in public. It could be a disaster."

"Don't worry. You just keep covered up with the baby blanket. You'll be fine!"

We ordered burgers and iced tea. Mom cut my burger in half for me so I could eat it while I fed Claire. But I still wasn't doing very well, so she took Claire from me for a burp, throwing the blanket on her shoulder just in time, handing her back for another round seconds before wailing would have surely ensued.

I got through my burger. It was a great burger, a memorable burger: bacon, cheddar, a big fresh tomato slice, the works. Claire got through her feeding. We spent several minutes in the restroom doing a complicated diaper change. Then, finally, we shopped.

I needed new pajamas. Something practical.

"I wish I could get these," I sighed, Eeyore-like, fingering some lovely peachy satin pajamas, the kind Myrna Loy would wear in a Thin Man movie.

"Why not?" Mom said. "They're not real satin, look at the price! Machine washable too! Life is short. And this color is so beautiful on you."

I bought them. I didn't wear them much, because they turned out to be a sort of unbreathable, man-made fabric that was way too warm. But the sight of them all shiny in my drawer was like the gentle and courtly Dr. Ottosen telling me to love myself. Only better, because it was Mom telling me to love myself. Just like she showed me that Northgate day that I really could take care of myself and my baby at the same time, that I really could buckle the car seat in if I swore a little and laughed a lot, that just because I had a baby didn't mean I didn't deserve a pair of impractical pajamas, the kind she must have known I would put on occasionally mainly for the pleasure of having Rus admire me in them for five minutes or so before removing them.

When Claire was born, a dozen years had passed since Ron died: since that terrible time when, for the first time in her life, Mom's customary lightness could not keep her buoyant. When, for a little while, she quietly drowned.

I have often wondered if that's when Alzheimer's disease saw its chance and went to work, even though it was another decade before she or we noticed the changes. Sort of like when a tree is mortally wounded during a season of fierce weather—an ice storm or a drought—and appears to recover, but inside, there's that weakness, that soft place, where illness or rot will some day set in.

But after she died, we didn't dwell on those dark days or on the many, many dark days that came later.

What happened after Mom died was something we could not have foreseen: after years and years, suddenly we were freed from dwelling on her daily diminishment, the slow, sap-leaking grief of it, and into this new space in our hearts came flooding all of our memories of the mom we'd known as children. Because we didn't have to make those dark, lonely visits anymore, we could dwell instead, at last, on how light she was.

It was an unexpected gift. The long years of conserving emotional energy were over. Now we could let go of hoarded feelings, we could cry and grieve and remember, like you're supposed to do after you lose your mother. For more than a decade, we'd been stuck in the cogs and wheels of losing her. Now she was lost and gone. Now we had a before and an after, like other bereaved people.

We had been missing her for so long already. Now, at last, we could say goodbye.

At her memorial service, we all got up and told stories about Mom. There were plenty to tell: Many variations on the crazy ski trip theme, including fond memories of Mom crouching in the snow next to our old station wagon, patiently tying together broken tire chains with shoelaces. Or the Mom-goes-off-to-college theme, featuring happy visions of her riding her bike to the University of Washington campus, unfazed by protest marches and sit-ins and unfazed by all the papers she had to write with all of us underfoot. Or travel tales, like Mom and Kristie going to Finland together and sitting in the sauna with distant cousins, who suddenly started thrashing themselves and their guests with bundles of birch twigs.

I pondered what I should tell.

I decided to go for a story with a little glamour to it.

The preamble: After college and fifteen months of working the lower rungs of Little, Brown and Company, I went to England to live with Dick, my future first husband, who was studying literature at Cambridge. I worked as a waitress at a popular American-style pizza restaurant. At the end of the school year, Mom came over and met me and we traveled through Europe on Eurail passes.

It was 1980. She was forty-nine; I was twenty-three. We had never in our lives spent a whole day, let alone three straight weeks, together without the rest of the family. But what I had hoped would be true, as we planned the trip, turned out to indeed be true: we wanted the same things from travel. When we weren't on the train, we wanted to be on foot, walking everywhere, sometimes with a destination and sometimes without one. We cared more about cafés and shops and atmosphere than checking off the tourist sights, though art was important to us. Stained glass and paintings, preferably rich in color and brushwork, moved us. Statues, crown jewels, ancient furniture—not so much. Good food was a pleasure but we didn't need it to be the best.

Our favorite stop of the trip was the Pension Mary-Flore, an old, family-run hotel in Nice with tall, balconied windows that reminded us of Matisse's paintings from his own days in Nice, those luscious paintings of windows full of blue sky and sea, curtains fluttering, shutters askew. We paid for the luxury of our own shower—and then realized it was, quite literally, in the room, sticking out from the wall like a light fixture. Not even a curtain around it. The floor was tile and there was a drain. But still, there was absolutely no way to take a shower without spraying the beds and everything else. And it made us laugh so hard that it took even longer to shower, which made even more of a mess.

We got a little better at it each day. We had no choice, after swimming in the salty Mediterranean, which we loved so much that we stayed on a few days, an act of sacrilege on the Eurail circuit.

Our last night in Nice, we decided to hop the train over to Monte Carlo for a little people watching. We showered ourselves—and our room—and then got as dressed up as we could: me in a twirly skirt, Mom in a strappy red sundress with a print of little white racehorses all over it. Her shoulders looked so sleek and tanned in that dress. Her hair was short and she was still dying it dark brown. She looked great and I could tell she felt great, too: excited and confident that it would be a memorable evening.

Mom knew more about Monte Carlo than I did, mostly from the movies and from following the story of Princess Grace. She wanted to see the Casino, she wanted to see elegant people and she wanted to have a drink at the Hotel de Paris, preferably champagne.

Monte Carlo on a summer evening sparkled. The hotel looked to us like an old palace, glittering at the top of the hill, limousines purring into the drive. We smoothed our hair and skirts and strolled purposefully up the steps, like we did this all the time.

Just as we reached the entrance, a limo pulled up and who should step out but Johnny Carson. He turned and saw us and flashed his big white Tonight Show smile, skimming it gently past me and resting it right on Mom. She smiled right back at him, matching him watt for watt, her eyes shining. Then he gave us a long wave and disappeared inside.

Mom was momentarily stunned. I took her arm and guided her into the bar.

"Two glasses of champagne," I said, and then we looked at each other and burst into laughter.

"It was just a smile," she said.

"Mom, he *wanted* you."

"The smile was enough."

"Mom, you look fabulous. I bet he's thinking about you right now."

"I'm just a miner's daughter from Butte, Montana."

"Yeah, and he's from Nebraska or somewhere, isn't he?"

"You bet he is. And that's the whole point, isn't it?"

"The point of what?"

"What makes life great. That a kid like him can become rich and famous and stay at the Hotel de Paris and a kid like me can grow up and have six kids of my own and put on a dress and smile at Johnny Carson and walk right in here and have a glass of champagne. Just like that!"

Just like that.

Just a miner's daughter, just a humble Clementine. At twenty-three, I never thought of my mom that way. At twenty-three, if you asked me to describe my mom, I would be more likely to tell you how proud I was that she had gone back to college and started a new life after her divorce. How different she was from the other moms, with their hospital guilds and teased hairdos. If I mentioned that she grew up in Butte, I would be more likely to talk about her high school stardom, her reputation as the braini- est girl in Butte High, the thick paragraph of accomplishments next to her name in the yearbook: band, art club, geometry award, trigonometry award, scholarship ribbon, senior council. I imagined Butte in the 1940s as a place of skating parties, proms, horseback rides in the country, not the place where my mom had been the daughter of a miner who dropped out of high school and did nothing but hard physical labor his whole life, except during the worst years of the Depression when there was no labor to do. It was later, as Alzheimer's pushed her brain back down those child- hood roads, that I finally understood how poor she'd been.

We toasted Johnny Carson. Then we strolled across the bluff to the

Café de Paris and dined outside under strings of starry lights, her smile still bright enough to light up all of Monte Carlo.

What I said at her memorial service was that Johnny Carson's smile was almost, *almost* as pretty as hers.

Mom died on March 7, 2006. She was not quite seventy-five. I still think about her every day. I wish she was here, I wish Alzheimer's had never happened. Of course. But I also feel so genuinely lucky that she was my mom. That I have memories like the night in Monte Carlo and the ski trips and her singing "I Feel Pretty" in the basement while she sorted laundry.

She was, as filmmakers like to say, an amazing source of natural light.

As for the darker parts of her life, especially her final years, writing helps, though sometimes I wish I were a scientist.

Participating in research helps, because then at least I'm helping the scientists.

But feeling helpful doesn't mean I don't still feel helpless.

Three years ago, I took part in a study that included a brain MRI: a Star Trek–like experience in which I lay down on a sort of conveyor belt that slid me into a tube that took pictures, mysteriously produced from a potion of magnetic fields and radio frequencies, of my brain. Rus filmed it, thinking that we might do something with it someday. All we've done so far is write "brain" on a videotape dated 1/9/2007.

I popped it in the player on my desk, just once, and looked at it.

The MRI image on the technician's computer screen was—disappointing. Underwhelming. It looked like any old black and white picture of a brain from a junior high science textbook. There were all the interesting pillowy shapes, some big, some small, some folded in accordion pleats, all arranged to fit perfectly inside a profile drawing of a human head. Then this first view morphed on the screen into many different views: making it more of a slide show than a textbook, but still redolent of darkened classrooms on sleepy afternoons.

"It's not just any brain, it's *my* brain," I tried to tell myself. "That's me in those pillows. Who I am. Right there." But it was too abstract.

Then I heard some audio on the tape. I turned it up. It was the MRI technician, talking to Rus.

"She has a beautiful brain," he said. "But you knew that."

I played it again, just to be sure.

A beautiful brain. As of 1/9/2007, I had a beautiful brain. It's nice to know. I think.

When Rus and I were filming interviews for *Quick Brown Fox* with Mom's Butte High classmates at their fifty-fifth reunion, the first thing one of them said about Mom was, "She had the most wonderful, wonderful brain." Not, "She was so smart," or "She was sure brainy," but, "She had the most wonderful brain." And I knew just what she meant: a brain that won trig and geometry prizes and painted vividly and loved literature; that later in life bounced back from tragedy, bought her first Eurail pass at forty-nine, put on a red sundress and set out for Monte Carlo—this was once a wonderful, wonderful brain. A beautiful brain.

According to the written report, the autopsy of Mom's brain showed "severe atrophy" in the temporal lobe and hippocampus, both essential to learning and memory. "Neuritic plaques," and "neurofibrillary tangles" were everywhere. Lewy bodies, another kind of brain plaque that may be related to Parkinson's disease, were "abundant" in the amygdala, where strong emotions are processed and remembered. The average healthy brain weighs three pounds; at death, hers weighed about 2.3 pounds. The report concludes: "The following processes contributed to the patient's dementia: Alzheimer's disease and Lewy body disease, amygdala predominant."

She was tested for the genetic marker that is associated with Alzheimer's disease, but in keeping with current research protocol, this result was not disclosed to us. If we decide we want to know, we would need to have the test done by a private laboratory.

People sometimes ask me if I do want to know whether Mom had the marker or whether I have it. The short answer is no, not unless there is something positive I can do with the information. It is hardly definitive: about one out of every three or four of us have this marker, known as the APOE4 allele, and about forty percent of people with Alzheimer's disease have it. In our mother's big family tree, there is not an overwhelmingly strong history of Alzheimer's disease: just Mom and one great-aunt. But if my children wanted to know, for example, or if I or they or Rus thought I was showing early signs of dementia, then maybe I would get tested. There are drugs you can take that are most effective in the early stages of Alzheimer's, drugs that can't stop the illness but may slow it.

Mom took one of those drugs for a while. We'll never know whether it made a difference, because we don't know how the disease would have progressed if she hadn't taken it. But during her steep, grim, late-stage descent, we looked back on some moments from those earlier Alzheimer's years as almost oasis-like.

I remember walking with her one sunny day along the south end of Lake Washington. We weren't talking much, which made me feel sad and guilty. I was in a dark, Alzheimer's-hating mood and I could not summon up the energy to talk; I couldn't bear the thought of having to explain some inane thing over and over again.

Suddenly Mom leaned over.

"Look at this rock!" she exclaimed.

"Where?" I didn't see it.

"Right here." She picked up a small, gray, absolutely ordinary beach rock, cradling it as if it were a robin's egg. She held it out to me, smiling. "Look at how round it is!"

"You're right, Mom." How could I disagree? "It is so perfectly round." She put the rock in her pocket. We walked on.

A few feet later she stopped and looked all around at the lake and the spring-green trees and the mountains and she sighed, contentedly.

"We live in such a beautiful place," she said. One of her stock lines, though she said it, as she always did, as if she'd never said it before and it was a completely new thought. But again, how could I disagree?

Then another stock statement, delivered with the same enthusiasm: "You know, all the trees were so small when I first moved here. Now look at them!"

This one always perplexed me a little. Hadn't there always been plenty of tall trees in Seattle?

Then one Sunday I saw a "Then and Now" photo spread in the *Seattle Times*. The point of it was how much our urban tree canopy has matured in the fifty or so years since the last big construction boom inside the city limits, and how the new trend of tearing down old ranch houses and modest bungalows and replacing them with either oversized mini-mansions or cheek-by-jowl townhomes was threatening the city's trees, many of which were planted after World War II. Which was right before Mom moved to Seattle. So she really did remember a time when all the streets were lined with saplings. And somehow, as Alzheimer's blocked off a few lanes here and cul-de-sacs there in her brain, she found herself continually revisiting that memory and appreciating how tall the tiny trees of her youth had become.

This often led her back to her "Nothing grew in Butte, Montana" riff. And so, moving along with her, I would find myself making the same circle: *We live in such a beautiful place. Look how the trees have grown in fifty years. Nothing grew in Butte, Montana.*

Can growing up in a place where nothing grew have been good for the body chemistry that fueled her brain? I wish I could send a team of scientists to Butte to find out.

And yet, there are so many toxic places in the world. And Mom has plenty of old friends from Butte who are doing just fine.

I ran into a few of them recently, at the University of Washington Alzheimer's Disease Research Center's luncheon honoring research volunteers. As far as I could tell, Jack and Frankie were still firmly in the control subject category. They began talking to another couple at our table who happened to have grown up in Great Falls. Before we knew it, the four of them were belting out the Montana state song: *"Tell me of that Treasure State, story always new, Tell of its beauties grand, and its hearts so true . . . "*

The couple they were singing with were retired Methodist ministers: the wife wading slowly into the middle waters of Alzheimer's where, though she could barely speak, the Montana state song came flowing back in a heartbeat.

Awards were given for the oldest research volunteer, who was 103; the volunteer who had done the most spinal taps—seven; the two volunteers who had been participating the longest—twenty-two years.

You realize, on a day like that, how very much company you have in the world. How very many families have been through this. Are going through this.

You realize the ripple effect.

Our neighbors had to take down an old tree recently, a Douglas fir between our driveway and their yard that had never looked well in all of the twenty years we've lived here, though it must have had a healthy youth to have grown so tall. Some long-ago sickness had burrowed deep into its heartwood, hammering away for years at its natural vigor, the way Alzheimer's took hold in Mom long before we knew it was there.

But the fir's gaunt branches always had an austere dignity, like a thin old man who was clearly once as dashing as Johnny Carson. And the birds loved its spacious perches.

The tree man climbed it, chainsaw in hand, and took down a few feet at a time. It took him all day. Our neighbor piled the branches in his yard. Up close, the branches looked healthy, brushy with green needles, not spindly and lonely, the way they had looked up on the tree, spaced so far apart.

The sight of such a tall tree coming down made passersby stop.

"It's been sick for a long time," people said.

"One big windstorm and it could've taken down that power line."

"I know the birds will miss it."

Now, from my office window, the street looks bare. A utility pole formerly sheltered by the tree is exposed and ugly. And the birds are circling, puzzling over whether to check out the chimneys or just head over to the park.

My brother and sisters and I are like that. We're never quite sure where to gather on birthdays and holidays. Our houses feel like saplings that aren't grown up yet. Too few branches. Not enough shade.

I think we just need the occasional good soaking rain. And time, lots of time. And plenty of light.

The End

Acknowledgments

My mother, Arlene, was with me every minute I spent writing this book. Though I will always wish her story had ended differently, I am honored to have written this version of it and I am so fortunate that she was my mom. I might not be a writer at all if not for the inspiration of Arlene's indomitable *sisu*—a Finnish word that in my mind means grit and pluck with a little humor thrown in.

My husband, Rustin, was my first and best reader. He loved me, encouraged me, fed me, took on way more than his share of everything and somehow kept the whole family's joie de vivre humming through not only the writing of this book but also the toughest years of Arlene's illness.

Our children, Claire and Nick, never wavered in their loving compassion for their grandmother and in their understanding of why I needed to write *Her Beautiful Brain*.

I am also forever grateful to my extended family, especially my sister Kristie, who read an early draft with a fine-toothed comb for historical accuracy, and my dad, Mike Hedreen, who let me interview him for two hours.

Thanks also to Nancy Nordhoff for founding Hedgebrook, an indescribably nurturing haven for women writers; to Goddard MFA advisors Michael Klein and Victoria Nelson for their inspiration, insight, and direction; to Goddard mates Isla McKetta, Priya Keefe, Karen Hugg, Ann Keeling, Natasha Oliver, Elizabeth Howard, and Ellen Welcker; to Hedgebrook role models Bishakha Datta, Irina Reyn, Yvette Heyliger, Ruth Ozeki, Claire Dederer, Barbara Howett, Loreen Lee,

Donna Miscolta, Allison Green, and Elizabeth Austen with an "e"; and to early readers, patient listeners, friends, and moral supporters Nancy Rinne, Anne Daley, Dana Robbins, Lisa Phillips, Lindsay Michel, Vicky Jamieson-Drake, Pat Duggan, Joe Unger, Ellen Cole, Dodi Fredericks, Kristine Forbes, Susan Rosenbaum, Susan Rava, David James Smith, Caroline Becker, Ellen Blaney, Elizabeth Austin with an "i," Holly Hughes, Mary Jane Knecht, Ron Reagan, Bonnie Vaughan, Carmen Ficarra, Lisa Moore, and Faith Conlon.

Thanks to the doctors and staff of the University of Washington Alzheimer's Disease Research Center, especially Drs. Murray Raskind, Elaine Peskind, James Leverenz, and Thomas Bird. Thanks to Kirsten Rohde, R.N., who first encouraged me to volunteer for research.

Thanks to the indomitable Keri Pollock and her colleagues at the Western and Central Washington chapter of the Alzheimer's Association.

Thanks to Women Make Movies, Northwest Film Forum, KCTS, Women in Film/Seattle, Greg Olson at the Seattle Art Museum, and the many individual donors who supported our 2004 film, *Quick Brown Fox: An Alzheimer's Story.*

Finally, thank you to Brooke Warner, Kamy Wicoff, and Caitlyn Levin of She Writes Press. I am so honored to be part of this new and exciting venture.

About the Author

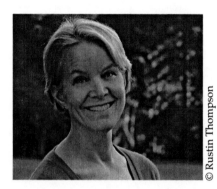

© Rustin Thompson

Ann Hedreen is a writer, filmmaker, teacher and voice of the radio podcast and blog, *The Restless Nest*. She and her husband Rustin Thompson own White Noise Productions. Together, they have made more than 100 films, many of which have been seen on PBS and other TV stations all over the world and some of which have won Emmys and other awards. They have two grown-up children and live in south Seattle.

Ann has an MFA from Goddard College and is an alumna of the Hedgebrook center for women writers. Her work has been published in *Seattle Metropolitan Magazine* ("Alzheimer's: Laughter and Forgetting," Society of Professional Journalists' First Place/Pacific Northwest winner for Science & Health reporting, 2012) *Courageous Creativity, Verbalist's Journal*, the *Pitkin Review*, the *Seattle Times*, the *Seattle Post-Intelligencer*, *Grist*, the *Sunday Observer* of Bombay, the *Galen Stone Review* and broadcast on NPR affiliate *KUOW*. She earned her B.A. at Wellesley College and began her career at the City News Bureau of Chicago.

Ann speaks and writes frequently about Alzheimer's disease and has volunteered as a control subject for many Alzheimer's studies. So far, she's undergone five spinal taps for the cause.

SELECTED TITLES FROM SHE WRITES PRESS

*She Writes Press is an independent publishing company
founded to serve women writers everywhere.
Visit us at www.shewritespress.com.*

Where Have I Been All My Life? A Journey Toward Love and Wholeness
by Cheryl Rice $16.95, 978-1-63152-917-7

Rice's universally relatable story of how her mother's sudden death launched her on a journey into the deepest parts of grief—and, ultimately, toward love and wholeness.

Pregnant Pause: A Memoir of Acceptance by Colleen Haggerty $16.95, 978-1-63152-923-8

Haggerty's candid story of how she overcame the pain of losing a leg at seventeen—and of terminating two pregnancies as a young woman—and went on to become a mother, despite her fears.

Americashire: A Field Guide to a Marriage by Jennifer Richardson $15.95, 978-1-938314-30-8

A couple's decision about whether or not to have a child plays out against the backdrop of their new home in the English countryside.

Splitting the Difference: A Heart-Shaped Memoir by Tré Miller-Rodríguez $19.95, 978-1-938314-20-9

When 34-year-old Tré Miller-Rodríguez's husband dies suddenly from a heart attack, her grief sends her on an unexpected journey that culminates in a reunion with the biological daughter she gave up at 18.

The Coconut Latitudes: Secrets, Storms, and Survival in the Caribbean by Rita Gardner $16.95, 978-1-63152-901-6

A haunting, lyrical memoir about a dysfunctional family's experiences in a reality far from the envisioned Eden—and the terrible cost of keeping secrets.

Four Funerals and a Wedding: Resilience in a Time of Grief by Jill Smolowe $16.95, 978-1-938314-72-8

When journalist Jill Smolowe lost four family members in less than two years, she turned to modern bereavement research for answers—and made some surprising discoveries.

CPSIA information can be obtained at www.ICGtesting.com
Printed in the USA
BVOW02s1907060814

361676BV00002B/7/P